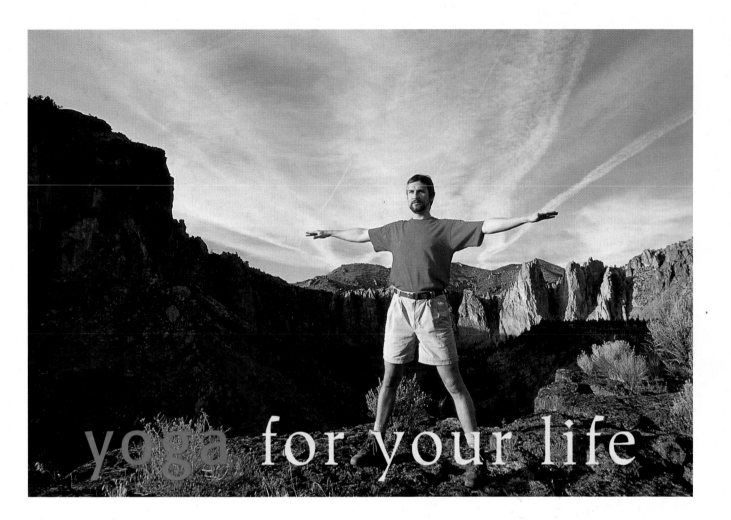

yoga for your life

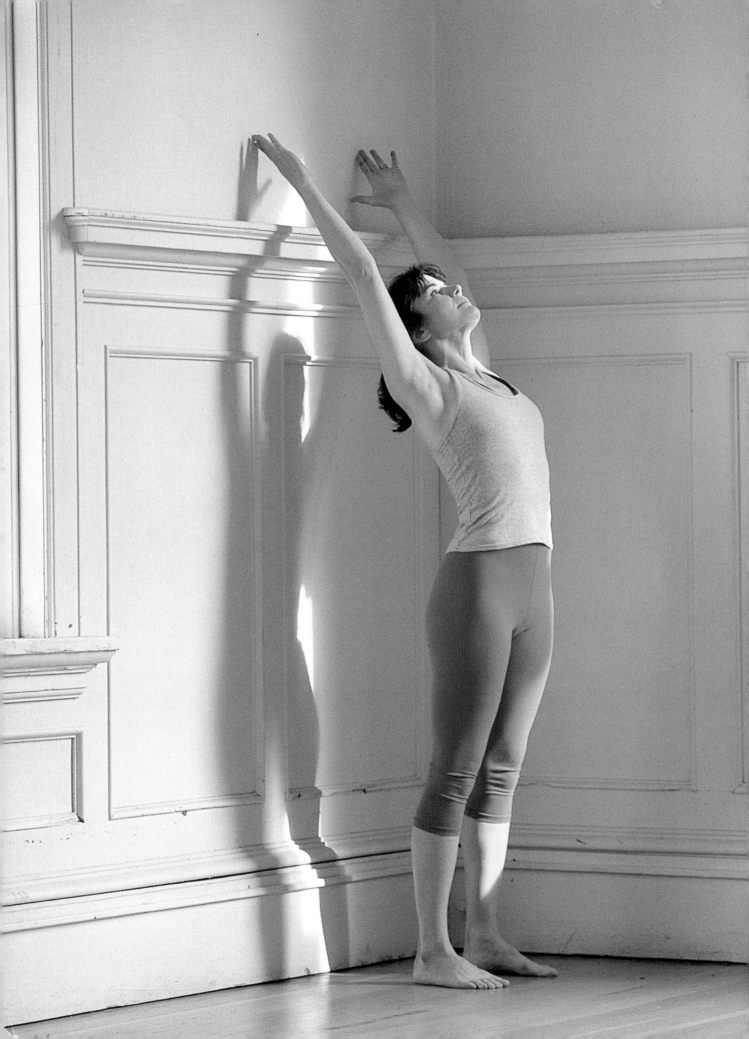

a practice manual of
breath and movement
for every body

yoga for your life

Margaret D. Pierce and Martin G. Pierce

BASED ON THE KRISHNAMACHARYA-DESIKACHAR APPROACH

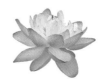

Photography by Barry Kaplan

RUDRA PRESS

PORTLAND OREGON

Printed in Canada

Rudra Press, PO Box 13390, Portland, Oregon 97213
Telephone: 503-235-0175
Telefax: 503-235-0909

Art direction and design by Bill Stanton
Photography by Barry Kaplan

Black and white photographs on pages 22, 30, 42, 54 and 70 are by Judy Kuniansky; on page 80, by Michael Romeo; on page 92, by Ann Borden; and on page 106, Mark Hill. Photo of ice skater on page 107 is provided by FPG International.

This book is not intended to replace expert medical advice. The authors and publisher urge you to verify the appropriateness of any procedure or exercise with your qualified health care professional. The authors and publisher disclaim any liability or loss, personal or otherwise, resulting from the procedures and information in this book.

Library of Congress Cataloging-in-Publication Data

Pierce, Margaret D.
    Yoga for your life : a practice manual of breath and movement for every body / by Margaret D. Pierce and Martin G. Pierce : photography by Barry Kaplan.
        p.   cm.
    ISBN 0-915801-60-4 : $20.00
    1. Yoga.   I. Pierce, Martin G.   II. Title
B132.Y6P49   1996
613.7'046—dc20   95-49675
                                              CIP

Printed in Canada

00 99 98 97   10 9 8 7 6 5 4

foreword

I am delighted that my longtime students and friends Margaret and Martin Pierce have written such a wonderful, practical manual on yoga—and more.

This book has been growing for many years. Margaret and I went over the first draft here in Madras in 1982. Since then, she and Martin have written many subsequent drafts.

Yoga for Your Life is the result of many years of learning, experimentation, analysis, and refinement. Martin and Margaret have worked out what they feel is the best way of teaching yoga to Westerners. They have tested it on their students. They have experimented to find better ways of explaining yoga poses and gearing them to what people really need.

Yoga for Your Life contains a carefully crafted series of lessons that builds safely and progressively. It is a friendly book, with numerous alternative suggestions. It becomes like a companion to the reader—especially as the reader moves to the special programs in the later part of the book.

Margaret and Martin's instruction is geared toward the beginning student, but really it is for everybody. The more one practices yoga, the more one appreciates the power of the most simple postures and breathing. And one doesn't have to wait until one is "advanced" to appreciate the tremendous benefits of meditation.

I wholeheartedly recommend this book to the beginning yoga student as well as to the experienced practitioner and teacher of yoga.

T.K.V. Desikachar
Madras 1995

contents

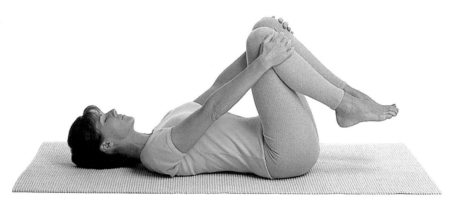

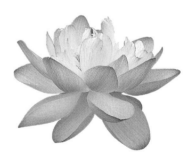

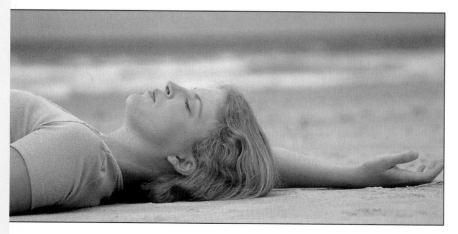

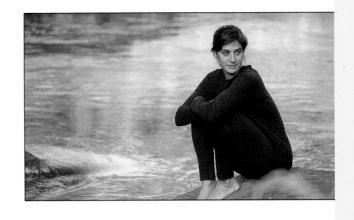

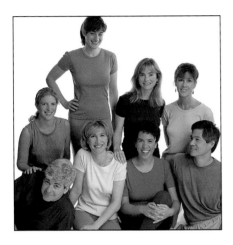

introduction

- A high-level executive closes his office door. He practices his "Short Relaxing Yoga Program" and emerges refreshed in the midst of a hectic day.

- A pregnant woman in labor lies in a hospital delivery room. Her eyes are closed, her breathing is slow and smooth, and she looks so peaceful and relaxed that her physician thinks for a moment that she is sleeping.

- A college student, in weight training, does a few yoga poses and then can bench press an additional fifteen pounds.

- An anxious health care professional goes to yoga classes for two nights before her Ph.D. oral exams. She is so relaxed that she "floats" through her test and calmly reads a magazine while she waits for her results.

- An internationally-known scholar practices yoga regularly, in whatever city or country she is visiting, to relieve the tension of a busy schedule and to keep what was once a severe back problem under control.

- An Episcopalian priest uses yoga as a means for spiritual growth.

- A busy executive, divorced and living alone, practices yoga poses every evening when she gets home, instead of reaching for the ice cream and cookies that she used to eat.

- A ten-year-old does several poses that are simple and fun, to help him concentrate in the classroom.

Each of these people is now or has been a student of ours. Our students come from all walks of life. Many are hard-driving professionals in high-pressure jobs. Others are busy parents with growing families to care for. We have taught yoga to very young children, to octogenarians, and to all ages in between. I, Margaret, regularly offer classes for pregnant women. We have even adapted poses for bedridden elderly or ill students.

We have been teaching yoga in Atlanta since 1973 at the Pierce Program center and as part of the physical education program of Emory University. During our years of teaching, we have seen yoga enrich thousands of lives and relieve a lot of pain and suffering.

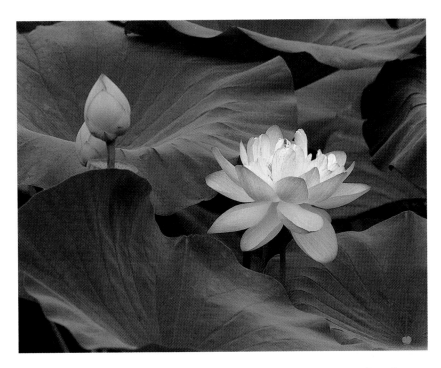

Neither one of us set out to become a yoga teacher. I, Martin, was a political science instructor at New York University, and I, Margaret, was a college student just back from two years of study in Vienna, Austria, and preparing for graduate school, when we each took our first yoga classes in the United States.

We have been fortunate to meet and study with an unusual man, T.K.V. Desikachar. Desikachar studied yoga with his father, T. Krishnamacharya, the greatest authority on yoga of his time and the man who taught many of the world's best-known yoga instructors. T. Krishnamacharya, in turn, learned from his father and other great teachers in a line that goes back at least 1,200 years. Desikachar transmitted this lineage of teaching and learning to us. Between us, we have made eighteen trips to India to study yoga. Teaching yoga has become our life's work. We love it and the many wonderful friends it brings us.

The yoga we practice and teach is in a tradition that focuses on the needs of the individual. The poses have ancient roots that we have adapted for our American students. We have written this book because many people who have heard of our yoga tradition have told us that they would like to study it— even though they live far from someone who teaches it. Many of our students and fellow practitioners have also asked for a book to supplement our teaching or to share with a friend.

Yoga for Your Life is a practical manual designed for a beginner to use at home. The lessons offer enough variations so that almost everyone can benefit by practicing them. You don't have to be very flexible or thin to practice yoga. You don't have to put yourself in "pretzel" poses to enjoy increased energy, vitality, strength, and flexibility. Our style of yoga adapts to an individual's needs—no matter who you are. It is a yoga for every body.

the great all-purpose exercise

Yoga is an ideal form of exercise for every body. Consider its many benefits:

• It is a great way to stay limber and energetic.

As an example, consider Don Payne. This seventy-year-old businessman had arthritis so badly that his doctor recommended him for full disability. Now, with yoga poses, he is able to work five or six days a week in a high-pressure job that requires spending long hours on his feet.

For our older students, such as eighty-seven-year-old Rachel Newberry, a retired school teacher, yoga offers a means to continue or resume the physical activities that they enjoyed in their youth. "At Christmas, I'm one of the oldest ones," Rachel says, "and the others are amazed that I can sit on the floor and scramble around giving out the presents. I can do most of the things I have been doing all my life."

• It is safe. There is no body strain.

Yoga is an amazingly gentle approach to exercise. Because the poses can be easily adapted to the individual's needs, and because we work with relaxed knees and elbows, the strains, sprains, and other injuries that can be unfortunate side effects of many forms of exercise rarely occur.

• It improves athletic performance.

Yoga is a perfect warm up—or cool down—for other forms of exercise. In addition, athletes we have taught report it improves their performance by helping them focus their minds and raise their energy levels.

Bobbi Patterson, an Episcopal priest, uses yoga to stretch out her hamstrings before playing squash. "But mainly I use it to focus better; I can be attentive to the ball and the game and let go of other things."

• It can go anywhere.

Ellen Mickiewicz is a professor at Duke University and a fellow at the Carter Center in Atlanta. An internationally-known scholar and expert on the media in the Soviet Union, she lectures all over the world. For her, this highly adaptable approach to yoga is the ideal form of exercise: "It is remarkably versatile and portable," she says. In London, Moscow, or Budapest, Ellen simply rolls out her mat in her hotel room, and she is ready to exercise.

• It can help you become more relaxed and focused.

Practicing yoga can help you handle other activities better. For instance, when you give a speech or make a presentation, you will be more effective if you are relaxed, calm, and strong. If you play golf, tennis, or another sport, you may find that your yoga practice helps you focus on the ball, relax the muscles that might restrict you, and put your energy exactly where you want it. If you are a parent with a crying or rebellious child, he or she will be more responsive and secure if you have learned to be strong but relaxed when you express and communicate.

• It can help you become more sensitive and aware.

Yoga may help you become more aware of the world around you and more sensitive to your own body. The leaves on a tree may seem more vibrant and colorful. You may hear more in a piece of music than you knew was there. You may see and appreciate your friends' and family's good qualities more and be less bothered by their annoying ones. Food may taste better. This does not mean that you will become a glutton. In fact, as you become more sensitive to your body, you may want to eat less. Simple, healthy foods often taste better after yoga so that the unhealthy, fat-laden fast foods become less attractive.

• It is suitable for everybody.

Children, adults, senior citizens, pregnant and postpartum women, bedridden people—we have taught them all and seen them all benefit from this remarkable approach to yoga.

a modern interpretation of
an ancient exercise

The yoga described in this book comes from an ancient tradition. Yet it is modern and scientific. Archaeologists have found 4,000 year old figurines in what appear to be yoga poses. Oral traditions, referring to yoga philosophy, breathing, and poses, date back at least 3,000 years.

Our teacher, T.K.V. Desikachar, traces his own family tradition back at least 1,200 years to the South Indian sage, Nathamuni. Our teacher's father, T. Krishnamacharya, who died in 1989 after celebrating his 100th birthday, was the foremost exponent of yoga of his day. He was an extraordinarily accomplished yogi and scholar, an innovative therapist and spiritual guide. When Martin first met him in 1972, he was yoga's most authoritative teacher.

In his youth, Desikachar turned away from his father's traditional teachings and pursued a Western-style education. He graduated first in his class as a structural engineer and went to work for a Danish firm. Later Desikachar realized the importance of his father's unique knowledge. He left engineering behind and studied with his father for 27 years until a few months before Krishnamacharya died. Although Krishnamacharya trained many teachers in his lifetime, it was Desikachar to whom he most thoroughly and systematically passed on his knowledge.

Krishnamacharya taught that yoga poses and breathing should be adapted to fit individual needs. This principle proved perfectly suited to his son's engineering mind. Each new physical or psychological complaint presented by a student offers a fresh challenge. Once Desikachar carefully analyzes the individual's problem and need, he adapts precisely the right poses to help solve it.

Adapting to Fit the Needs of Each Individual

This approach is unique in that we constantly adapt ancient poses to make them fresh and relevant to the demands of today's fast-paced world. We change and combine poses (*asanas*), breathing (*pranayama*), and other yoga techniques to fit the large variety of individual needs. The main characteristics of this yoga tradition are:

• **It emphasizes breathing with movement.**

Students learn how to use their breath in yoga poses to promote balanced, relaxed energy and focused concentration. Proper breathing in poses strengthens you and increases your energy. If you feel anxious, angry, or unfocused, it can help you find your strong, calm inner self. As you move and breathe, your feelings about life often become more positive. Problems seem less burdensome as you glimpse the "big picture" of your life.

• **It adapts poses to your individual needs.**

Because one person's ideal workout may be someone else's pulled muscle or sprained knee, we try to tailor poses so they are right for your body type, muscle strength, and conditioning. We start from where people are. Rather than ask people to conform to an ideal postural form, our tradition makes poses conform to the needs of the individual.

A forward bend can gently limber up the new mother who stands beside her hospital bed and bends over only far enough to put her hands on the bed. The same pose can help an athlete work up a sweat and strenuously work his back—if he holds a thick dowel at arm's length. Another person might stay bent over and exhale slowly in the forward bend to relieve muscle spasms in her back.

Just as we adapt yoga to your particular needs, we also adapt it to your changing day-to-day needs. For example, if you are feeling tired in the afternoon and you know you have a busy evening ahead, you can lie down and do some arm movements for relaxation and then a simple arch for relaxed energy. If, on the other hand, you are all keyed up but it is bedtime, you can do a slightly different set of poses to help you sleep. There are poses to relieve anxiety and focus your mind before an exam or a board meeting, and poses to relieve depression after a disappointing day. You can do poses to feel rested, poses to work up a sweat, and many more.

Letting Out A Well-Kept Secret

You may not be familiar with this individualized approach to yoga poses, breathing, and meditation. Desikachar teaches through private lessons and has always preferred to work closely with a few people rather than superficially with many. It takes years, a lifetime, to train in this ever-changing tradition. That is why this yoga tradition, unfortunately, resembles something of a well-kept secret.

This approach to yoga has enormous potential for improving your daily life, in both quiet and dramatic ways. We wish it were as well-known and as accessible as aerobics or weight training. This is why we have taken many of our most helpful yoga poses and put them into an easily understood progressive eight-lesson format and then added eight special-purpose programs. We have seen time and again the many benefits that this approach offers. We want to let this well-kept secret work for you.

how to make yoga work for you

Yoga can help you take care of yourself! It is different from other kinds of exercise that emphasize your performance. Yoga helps you find inner as well as physical strength. In aerobics classes you move to exciting music and check yourself in a mirror. In yoga you do not need to worry about how you look. You are concerned about how you *feel*. You discover the peace and quiet available inside you. You will close your eyes during most of the poses to bring your awareness inward.

We have all learned to compete in school, in business, or in sports. Yoga helps you focus inward to discover who you are and what you want to be, rather than what the world is trying to make you do. Yoga helps you find a relaxed energy in your own mind and body.

For thousands of years, people who have practiced yoga have learned that we waste much of our energy. The problem starts with our minds, which produce a constant stream of thoughts; sometimes it seems as if our minds are out of control. Instead of staying focused on one thing, we are subject to a constant flow of thoughts. We wonder: "How can I do everything I need to do today?" and then start to make a mental list. We think: "I am happy about this; I'm worried about that." This dance of thoughts keeps us from concentrating and thinking clearly about any one thing. (If you don't believe this, just stop reading this book for a couple of minutes and try to envision your mind as calm and quiet. Note all the thoughts that pass through your head.) Without our even knowing it, this constant stream of ideas puts tension into our bodies—sometimes to the point of becoming ill.

The purpose of yoga is to quiet our minds so that our mental energy can go where we want it to. This allows us to focus on what we choose to concentrate on. This is called "one-pointed concentration." When you calm your mind by doing yoga, you also calm your body. You may realize that all those exciting, interesting, or worrisome thoughts were agitating and tensing your body. As the yoga poses slow you down, you become more relaxed.

Through yoga you also may discover that you have more strength and energy than you realized. The constant flow of your thoughts, muscular tensions, and other physical stresses use up an enormous amount of your energy. If you can relax and focus your energy, it is available for other purposes. You can be calm, quiet, and strong—physically and emotionally. You can become aware of a source of spiritual strength within you.

Yoga is different from other exercise, and you need to do it differently if it is going to work for you. Here are some principles to follow as you practice yoga:

To Gain Avoid Pain

Yoga should feel good. Elsewhere you might have heard: "No pain no gain." Yoga does not work like this. If you are to gain from yoga, you should avoid pain. Some exercise programs urge you to push yourself "until it hurts," but our approach does the opposite. In yoga, pain rarely brings gain. If something hurts, that means your exquisitely efficient nervous system is telling you something is wrong. You are about to injure yourself—or maybe you already have.

Forcing yourself through pain can prevent you from stretching and relaxing. When a movement causes pain, your muscles involuntarily tighten to protect themselves, and you may wind up tenser than before or you may even injure yourself.

If you feel pain during a pose, it probably means that the pose is not right for you, you have pushed too hard, or you have done too many repetitions. Try to find a way to adapt the pose or decrease the number of repetitions, or drop the pose altogether.

Take A Holiday from Stress and Competition

"Push a little harder!" "Come on, just one more! You can do it!" In the past you may have pushed yourself to the limit as you listened to such exhortations from a friend, a coach, or your own inner judge. Try to forget them while doing yoga.

Yoga helps you become more aware of what is right for you. Just because someone else can do a pose does not mean that you should do it. Avoid competing with yourself. Just because you could touch your toes yesterday does not mean you have to touch your toes today. Yesterday you may have been relaxed and rested. Today, perhaps your back and legs are tense and you need to move gradually into a stretch.

Be Relaxed and Alert as You Work Out

Several years ago, a reporter commented on the winner of a new world's record in the 200 meter dash: "He was the most relaxed runner." Whether the announcer knew it or not, he was saying that the winner had demonstrated a yoga principle. In a race that was won by hundredths of a second, the runner needed to put all his strength into the muscles that were pushing him to the finish line. He could not afford to waste energy in any other muscles. So he relaxed and won!

The traditional definition of a yoga pose or *asana* is a posture in which you are strong, alert, and relaxed. This means that you use just the muscles you need and no others. It also means you can work hard but without pushing beyond your limit.

There are many ways of relaxing. You can doze in the sun, lie in a sauna, or have a beer, but because you are not alert, you are not doing yoga.

You can push yourself to your physical limit by running, lifting weights, or swimming. But if you are not comfortable, if your exercise is not relaxed, you are not doing yoga.

Alertness means that as you do these poses, you keep your attention on your breath and on how your body feels. You learn to keep your breath flowing smoothly and evenly, with pauses after inhalations and exhalations. When you cannot do this, you will know that you are pushing yourself too hard or too fast. Relaxing means that you let go of any areas that you don't need to work—as the record-setting runner did. Working in this way, you protect yourself from injury and you focus your energy where it is needed.

Develop Your Mental Capacities

Yoga poses are designed to focus your mind and help you be more aware. Each pose is not only a physical posture, it is also a gentle mental discipline. When you do a yoga pose, you pay attention to what you are feeling and how you are moving. You learn to make subtle adjustments so that the pose works better for you. As you do this, the poses become exercises in pleasurable mental focus.

As you practice, your mind may stray to something interesting or bothersome in your life. We urge you not to chastise yourself for letting your thoughts wander. It happens to all of us. Just accept it, and gently bring your attention back to your breath and the pose.

As your body relaxes, your mind automatically slows down. Instead of thinking of many things at once, you can focus on the most important ones. Fewer thoughts going through your head leaves room for creative thinking. You may find the answer to a question you had been struggling with. You may suddenly say, "Oh yes, it's so simple. Why didn't I see that before?"

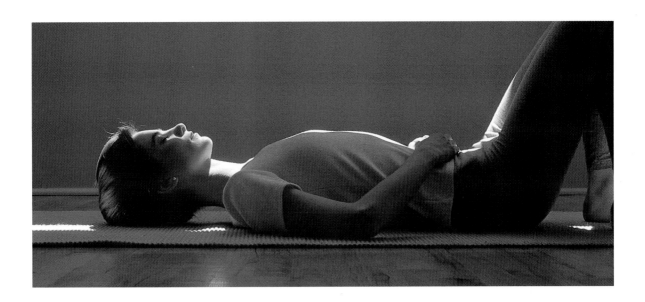

Discover Your Inner Self

Within each of us is a source of strength, mental clarity, and peace. The highest purpose of yoga is to find this inner source. Unfortunately, much of the time we may not be aware of this source. We may, in fact, not know who we truly are. Too often our minds are filled with a stream of thoughts that hold our attention, but in the long run may not be terribly important.

Yoga helps us eliminate some of the clutter and incessant chatter from our minds. Slow breathing not only can relax our bodies, it can quiet our minds. Recent medical studies suggest that deep, slow yoga breathing changes your body's chemistry and your nervous system. Following our instructions for breathing should help you relax and feel more peaceful. The poses help us focus on one thing instead of scattering our attention on many. When we calm our minds, we make space for the awareness of who we really are. We may become more conscious of our true Self, which an overly active mind conceals.

We have watched many people use yoga to change and become aware of something deeper and more important. They may call it the Real, the Self, the Source, Being, Brahman, Allah, God, Awareness, or they may prefer not to give it any name. What it is called does not matter.

What does matter is the inner growth that comes through yoga—a greater sense of inner calm, happiness, and an increase in caring and compassion for those around us. This is something worth doing a little yoga for every day.

how to use this practice manual

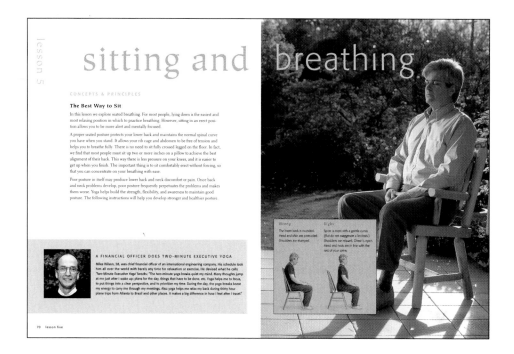

The Progressive Eight-Lesson Series

This book is designed to help you practice yoga on your own, even if you have not done yoga before. We present eight lessons that will take you from beginning level to more advanced poses and breathing. The lessons form a progressive series. The first few lessons emphasize relaxation, basic breathing, and simple movement patterns. The later lessons provide more strenuous and demanding poses that energize your body and focus your mind. We encourage you to follow the sequence of poses given. We hope you will move step-by-step through the lessons. Please do not skip to the more challenging lessons—even if you have practiced yoga before. Take the time to master the earlier lessons so that you benefit from the more demanding poses in later lessons and ensure that you do not injure yourself.

Each lesson starts with a Concepts & Principles section, where we expand on some of the basic principles of yoga movement and breathing. Explanations or some simple exercises help you to understand these principles in greater detail.

Next, there is step-by-step instruction through the lesson. Follow the sequence of poses and directions as you practice them for the first time. Spend at least 5-7 days on each lesson to master it before moving on. By practicing several times a week, you should gain the strength, stamina, and flexibility to become prepared for the next lesson containing more advanced work. You may find that you will want to work at a slower pace; you may want to practice each lesson for a few weeks before progressing. That is just fine. You set the pace that is best for you. Remember, in yoga we do not compete, even with ourselves.

Instructions and Pose Numbers

For each pose, the steps of the instructions are numbered; these numbers are keyed to the photographs to help you easily match instructions to the pictures as you practice. Often we give tips for adapting the pose. These are indicated with an arrow.

In addition, each pose is given a two-part number. For example, the third pose in Lesson Two is called "2.3 Triangle". The first number indicates the lesson in which the pose's instructions are first given. The second number is the sequence number within the lesson. In subsequent lessons, poses are referred to by their lesson/sequence numbers, so that you can find the instructions quickly if you need to refresh your memory.

PICTURE NUMBERS KEYED TO
INSTRUCTIONS HELP YOU
FOLLOW EASILY.

ARROW TIPS HELP YOU
ADAPT THE POSE TO YOUR
NEEDS.

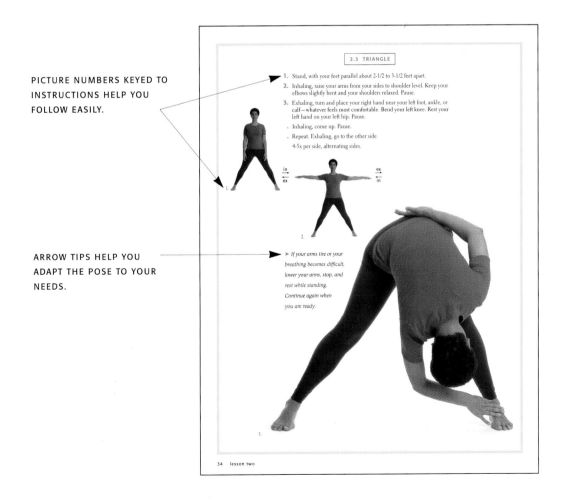

2.3 TRIANGLE

1. Stand, with your feet parallel about 2-1/2 to 3-1/2 feet apart.

2. Inhaling, raise your arms from your sides to shoulder level. Keep your elbows slightly bent and your shoulders relaxed. Pause.

3. Exhaling, turn and place your right hand near your left foot, ankle, or calf—whatever feels most comfortable. Bend your left knee. Rest your left hand on your left hip. Pause.

. Inhaling, come up. Pause.

. Repeat. Exhaling, go to the other side.

4-5x per side, alternating sides.

▶ If your arms tire or your breathing becomes difficult, lower your arms, stop, and rest while standing. Continue again when you are ready.

34 lesson two

Special Programs

Once you have worked your way through the eight-lesson progressive series, you can experiment with the special purpose programs later in the book. You might enjoy a vigorous work-out, a short relaxing sequence, an early morning wake-up, or a sequence for going to sleep. You might want to use yoga to help you warm-up before or cool-down after your regular exercise program. You can choose special programs to fit your own needs. Of course, you can go back to any one of the eight lessons, and do them again and again. The beauty of yoga is that each time you practice you learn something more about yourself, and you gain the benefits of increased relaxation, vitality, and mental focus.

Where to Practice

You can practice and enjoy yoga almost anywhere. We have practiced on rocky hiking trails in the mountains, in the far corner of an airport while waiting for a late plane, on secluded tropical beaches, and amidst a clutter of open suitcases with Christmas celebration resounding in the next room.

You will get more out of your yoga, though, if you practice somewhere where you are not distracted. A clean, neat, uncluttered, and quiet space with subdued lighting is best. Practice on a firm, thick carpet or mat. Many beginning yoga students do not realize that over time they can bruise themselves if they use too little padding. So please use a mat or rug that is a little thicker than you think you need.

When to Practice

For many people the best time to practice is first thing in the morning, before even fully waking up. If you start your day with yoga, it will wake you up, and you may find that you do not need a cup of coffee to get going. You may discover that you have more stamina and that you can concentrate and relax more easily during the rest of the day.

Many people like to practice before lunch, as a healthy midday pick-me-up. Afterward they feel more alert. Another good time to practice is before your evening meal. Then the poses may help you relax from the pressures of your day, renew your energy, and enable you to sleep more easily and deeply later on.

Some people have no time to practice except late in the evening, just before bedtime. If you cannot manage any other time, do it then, although you may find it hard to be attentive to your breath and movements when you are tired. If you do some relaxing poses with slow exhalations on the floor or bed, you may actually sleep better. But if you do the more energizing poses late at night, they may keep you from sleeping afterward.

Adapting Yoga Poses to Your Body

One of the benefits of this yoga tradition is that the poses can be adapted in an infinite number of ways to fit the individual's needs. In this book, we offer as many choices as possible to meet your needs. You can choose not only the pose but the way of doing the pose that is best for you. If a certain pose does not feel right or might possibly injure you, suggestions are given for a different variation or pose. Often, an adaptation box shows you how to change the exercise for your requirements. Sometimes slight changes in a pose help you work harder or less hard if you have a problem with it.

The programs presented are based on our combined forty-four years of teaching experience to the "average" person's needs in a group class. We include many ways of varying yoga poses, but obviously we cannot foresee all the needs of everyone who reads this book. Even if we tried to, we would have to show so many pose variations that the book would be extremely long and confusing.

You are not average—nobody is. You have your individual strengths and limitations. These lessons will help you to get started and practice. If you want to get the most out of yoga—especially if you have serious pains or ailments—we urge you to find an experienced, capable teacher who can adapt the poses and breathing specifically to your needs. Since we are not physically present with you to guide you into the safest and most helpful poses, please consult a competent teacher or your doctor about a pose *before doing it* if you are at all doubtful about it. If you encounter such a pose and want to continue doing a program, skip it and substitute a pose you feel comfortable with.

Practice and Experiment

The benefits of yoga practice are cumulative. If you practice properly you should feel better at the end of each session. If you can sustain your practice over a long period, you should feel a still greater benefit. It is not just that you become stronger or that you may be able to stretch and assume positions that you once thought were beyond you. Yoga retrains your mind and your nervous system, so that you learn to relax much more quickly. As you continue with yoga, you should gain a gradual sense of your own inner strength. You should find it easier to be the strong and focused person you really are.

Experiment with the poses. Enjoy the feeling of combining slow breathing with slow movement. Find the programs that best suit you and your needs. Become more aware of those needs through yoga. Be patient. Enjoy your new strength, flexibility, stamina, and ability to focus. And remember that according to the ancient sage, Patanjali, the definition of yoga is "to stop the whirlings of the mind." Yoga is far more than practicing acrobatic feats. It vitally links your body, breath, mind, and spirit.

We hope you enjoy the exploration.

breathing

Breathing is central to yoga. Your breath is the connection between your body and your mind. By calming your breath, you can relax your body and mind more deeply. Yoga breathing can increase your energy and open you to greater spiritual awareness. To help you understand the basics of yoga breathing, we'll start with a short relaxing exercise. As you practice, you will start to feel the effects for yourself. Let's begin!

• First lie down on a thick mat, carpet, or a firm bed. Rest with your legs comfortably apart. Place your arms about one foot from your sides, palms turned up. Relax your body onto the floor.

• Next, place one hand on your lower abdomen, the other on the lower part of your chest. Use your hands to feel your chest and abdomen move as you breathe. Notice the gentle expansions and contractions as your body moves with your breath.

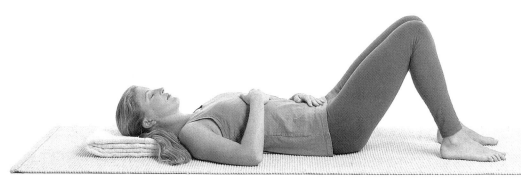

You may want to put a small pillow under your head and neck. If your lower back feels tense, put pillows under your knees or simply bend your knees and place your feet flat on the floor.

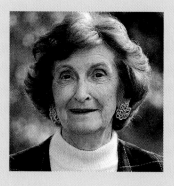

AN OVER-80 KEEPS HER SPIRIT AND BODY UP

Rachel Newberry, 87, taught Sunday School in Lizella, Georgia, for forty-seven years. When she retired, her church declared a Rachel Newberry Day: "Yoga keeps me supple, comfortable, and able to do things that others of my age can't. I can do most of the things I have been doing all my life. I haven't slowed down. Yoga is like a prayer. I do it with a great feeling of praise and thankfulness. Breathing in helps me to be conscious of receiving from everybody and everything that has ever been a part of my life. Breathing out gives me a sense of trying to give back something I have received. When I finish I am ready to say 'amen.'"

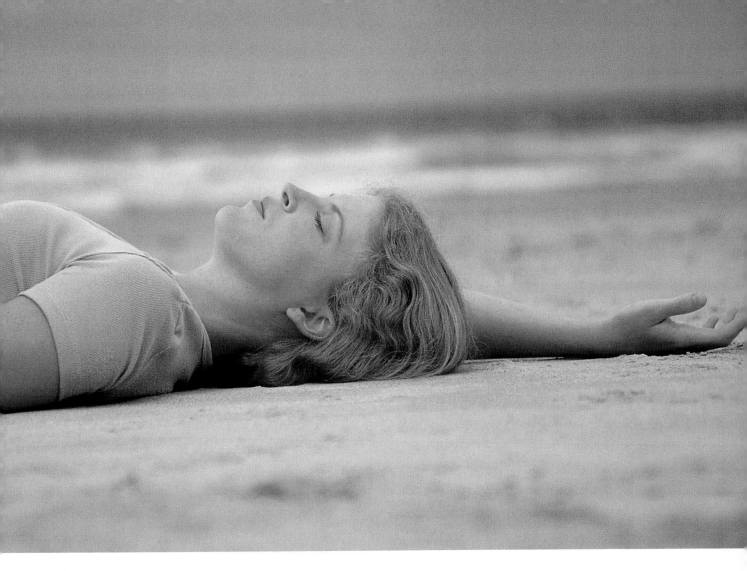

- Close your eyes and mouth.

- Inhale slowly, gently expanding through your rib cage or abdomen, whichever is more comfortable for you.

- Pause one or two seconds. Pausing after each inhalation and each exhalation will bring you a deeper sense of calmness and relaxation. These pauses will increase your concentration and awareness of your body.

- Exhale slowly, gently contracting your abdominal muscles.

- Pause one or two seconds.

- Inhale slowly, gently expanding.

- For the next 5 minutes, continue to breathe slowly, smoothly, and comfortably without forcing your breath in any way. Make sure your exhalation is the same length or a little longer than your inhalation.

- When you are done, release conscious control of your breathing. Notice how you feel. Is your body more relaxed? Are your thoughts more quiet?

Following the Poses in the Photographs

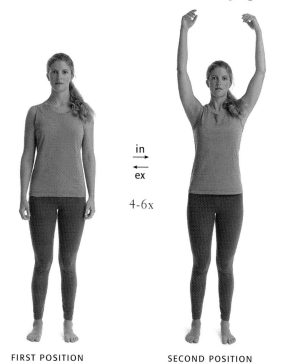

FIRST POSITION   SECOND POSITION

All of the movements in the book will be shown like this:

The arrows ⟶ indicate the movement and the breathing involved with the movement.

"in" means Inhale as you move from the initial FIRST position to the SECOND position.

"ex" means Exhale as you move from the SECOND position BACK to the FIRST position.

"x" means times. Here, we suggest that you raise and lower your arms 4-6 times.

How to Breathe

To breathe in the most relaxing way, close your mouth and breathe through your nose. Make a very slight, quiet sound with your throat. This hushed sound helps you better control the flow of your breath. Keep your breath slow and smooth, and focus your attention inward.

Listen to the sound of your breath. The sound should be constant and unwavering. Make sure that you inhale and exhale at a consistent rate. Avoid letting air rush in loudly at the beginning of your inhalation. Try not to breathe out so quickly at the start of your exhalation that you have to strain to complete it.

Avoid even the slightest strain in your breathing. If at any time, in a breathing exercise or while doing a pose, you strain or gasp for breath, you will know that you are pushing yourself too hard. Find a steady, comfortable rhythm. Feel the flow and become attuned to the soft, gentle sound of your breath.

Number of Repetitions

We suggest a number of repetitions for each pose. If you do too few repetitions, you may not become as deeply focused, or you may not stretch and strengthen yourself as much. If you do too many, the additional repetitions may fatigue you, or you may hurt yourself. After practicing the programs for a while you will get a feeling for whether you want to do more or fewer repetitions than we indicate. The number may vary from day to day. In general, try doing at least 4 and usually no more than 8 repetitions.

Eyes Opened or Closed?

To focus your attention inward, keep your eyes closed when you do lying, kneeling, or sitting poses. When you do standing poses, keep your eyes open, as you need, in order to maintain your balance.

Let's begin with the first lesson!

the lesson

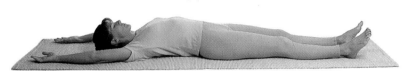

1.1 ARM RAISE

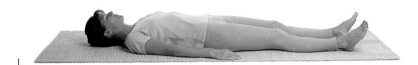

1.

ex ↑ ↓ in

2.

1. Lie comfortably on the floor. Place your arms alongside you with your palms down. Relax.

2. Inhaling, raise your arms forward and over your head. Place your hands onto the floor behind you. Pause.

1. Exhaling, lower your arms back down beside you. Pause. Then begin again with your next inhalation.

6-8x

➤ *Place a small pillow under your head and neck as needed. If your lower back feels tense, bend your knees and place your feet flat on the floor.*

1.2 UPWARD LEG AND OUTWARD ARMS STRETCH

1. Lie on your back. Place your left foot flat on the floor, with your right knee to your chest, your right hand on your right knee, and your left hand on your shin.

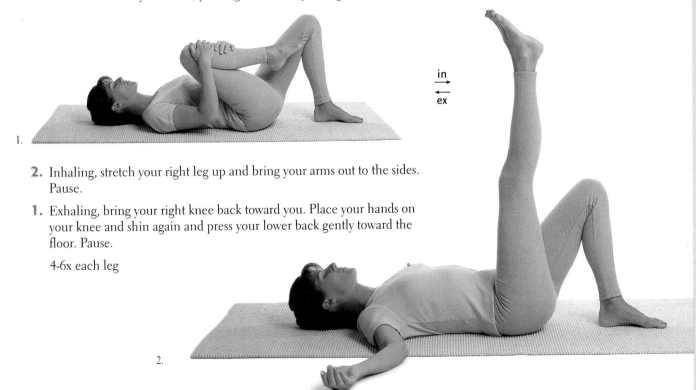

in
→
←
ex

1.

2. Inhaling, stretch your right leg up and bring your arms out to the sides. Pause.

1. Exhaling, bring your right knee back toward you. Place your hands on your knee and shin again and press your lower back gently toward the floor. Pause.

4-6x each leg

2.

➤ *If this pose is difficult for you, place a small pillow under your head and/or hips.*

1. Lie on your back with your feet flat on the floor. Place your feet about 6 to 18 inches apart at a comfortable distance from your hips. Place your arms close to your sides, palms down.

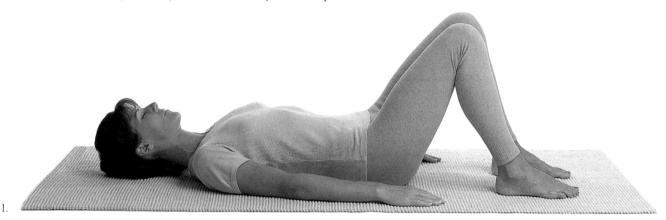

1.

ex ↑ ↓ in

2. Inhaling, slowly raise your hips off the floor, bringing your arms over your head onto the floor behind you. Keep your elbows slightly bent. Pause.

• Exhale while keeping your hips off the floor. Pause. Inhaling, raise your hips a little higher. Pause.

1. Exhaling, lower your arms and hips back to the floor.

4-6x

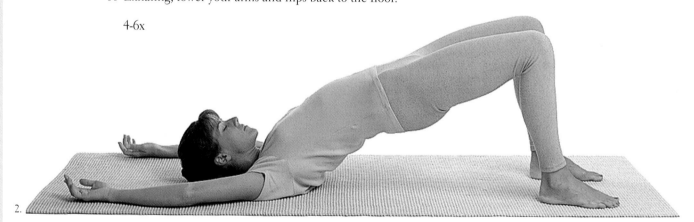

2.

1. Stand with your feet parallel, 6 to 12 inches apart.
2. Inhaling, raise your arms from the front. Pause with your arms over your head.

➤ If you can't touch the floor, if you have a back or sinus problem, if you are prone to headaches, or if this pose makes you dizzy, practice this and other forward bends to a chair (see the adaptation box in Lesson 2).

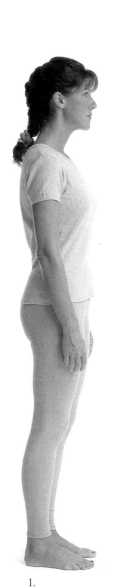

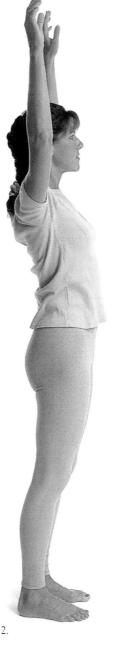

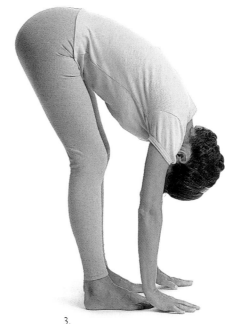

in
→
←
ex

ex
→
←
in

1.

2.

3.

3. Exhaling, bend forward. Allow your knees and elbows to bend slightly, and keep your arms and fingers relaxed. Pause.

2. Inhaling, come up keeping your knees slightly bent. Lead with your chest and your arms relaxed. Pause.

1. Exhaling, lower your arms to your sides.

5-6x

1.5 KNEES TO CHEST POSE

1. Bring your knees to your chest. Place your hands on or near your knees.

2. Inhaling, guide your knees away from you as you straighten your elbows. Pause.

1. Exhaling, bring your knees gently toward you. Pause.

4-6x.

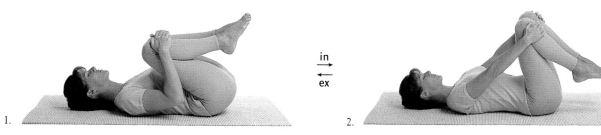

1.   in →   2.
                  ← ex

➤ *Place your hands on your knees such that your arms and shoulders remain relaxed. Can you breathe and move more easily with your knees together, well apart, or somewhere in between?*

1.6 LYING TWIST WITH BOTH KNEES BENT

1. Lie on your back. Bend your knees and place your feet flat on the floor 2 to 4 inches apart. Relax your arms out to the sides slightly below shoulder level, palms up.

2. Exhaling, bring your knees over to your right. Pause. Keep the right edges of your feet on the floor. Try to keep your left shoulder on the floor.

1. Inhaling, bring your knees back up to the original **(1)** position. Pause.

4-5x per side, alternating sides.

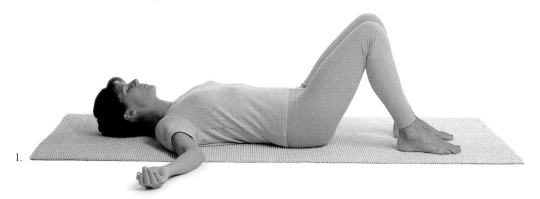

1.

in ↑ ↓ex

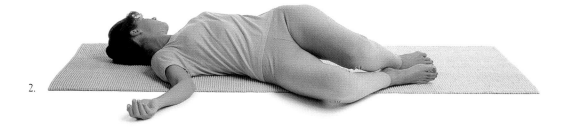

2.

28   lesson one

- Kneel with your knees slightly apart. Place your hands flat on the floor about shoulder width apart, wrists just slightly ahead of your shoulders.

1. Exhaling, move your hips partially or all the way back; bend your arms and relax your head onto or close to the floor. Pause.

2. Inhaling, move forward while slowly arching your back down and tilting your head comfortably back. Pause.

6-8x

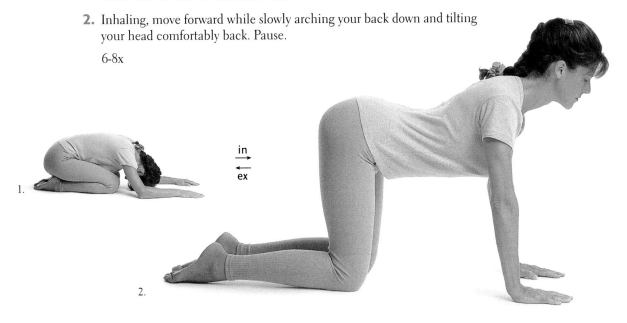

in
←
ex

1.

2.

1.8 LYING REST WITH FOCUSED BREATHING

- Lie comfortably on your back. Place your legs far enough apart so your hips and legs can be very relaxed.

- Place your arms by your sides about 12 inches away from your body, palms up. Close your eyes.

- Relax your body as you take 10-12 breaths. Try to make your exhalation longer than your inhalation. With each exhalation relax your face and eyes. Bring your attention more and more deeply inward with each breath.

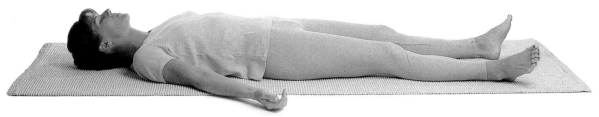

➤ *If your head tips back or your neck feels strained, place a small pillow under your head and neck.*

➤ *If your lower back feels tense, place a wide cushion under your knees. Or you can put your lower legs comfortably apart on a chair with your knees bent.*

➤ *If these positions are not convenient, simply bend your knees with your feet flat on the floor.*

Rest for 2 minutes.

breath in

CONCEPTS & PRINCIPLES

In Lesson One, you experienced the basic principles of yoga breathing. Now we'll look at how to become more aware of your breath and how to integrate your breath with your movement in all the yoga poses.

Refine Your Breathing

This next short exercise will help you attune yourself further to your breath. Review the breathing tips given in Lesson One before you start this exercise.

- Lie down comfortably and close your eyes.

- Breathe smoothly and evenly, gradually lengthening your breath.

- For the next 6 to 8 breaths find the longest breathing pace that you can comfortably sustain while still breathing smoothly. Mentally count the length of the breath. (Use one second for each count.) You may be able to inhale for 4 counts and exhale for 4 counts. Or perhaps you can comfortably inhale 6 counts and exhale 8 counts, or longer. The particular count doesn't matter. Just get to know your breath.

- Establish a consistent even rhythm.

- Stop counting the length of the breath, but continue to breathe at your deepest, most relaxed rate for 12 breaths.

- When you are done, release control of your breathing. Become aware of how you feel.

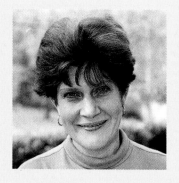

SHE EXCHANGED SMOKING FOR YOGA

Katie Teel, 45, an editor and writer, admits she was addicted to nicotine. She quit smoking several times but always started back: "This last time, I used yoga to quit. Now it has been more than thirteen years since I last smoked. Yoga gives me the same meditative in-and-out breathing that I got from smoking. When you smoke, part of what calms you is taking in air and breathing it out. It sounds funny because you're taking in horrible smoke, but you get addicted to the movement of the breath. I used to smoke when I worked, because I became mentally excited. I wanted to do something so that I could concentrate. Now I do yoga to rechannel my energy."

movement

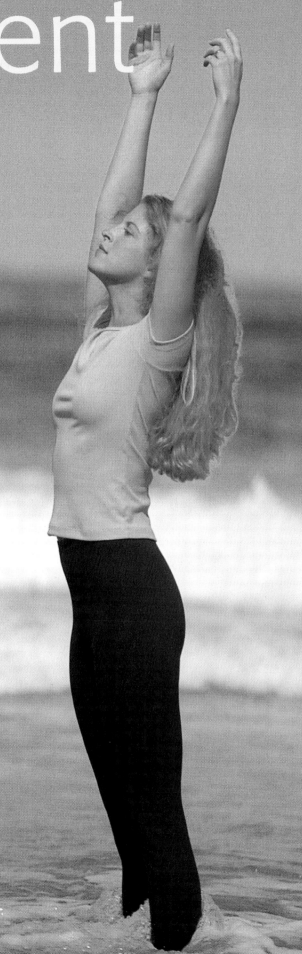

Breathing with Movement

In yoga, you will learn to coordinate your breathing with your movement. For instance, in the Arm Raise you inhale as you raise your arms, and exhale as you lower your arms. All the poses in this book have both inhalation movements and exhalation movements. As you coordinate your movements with slow, smooth breathing and pauses, your attention goes deeply inward. You focus your mind, thereby linking it to your breath and movements.

Each movement should take about 4-10 seconds, using the full length of your breath to complete it. Your exhalation should be the same length or somewhat longer than your inhalation. At first you may find that your breath is short, maybe you can comfortably breathe 4 seconds during each inhalation and exhalation. That's fine. Just try to coordinate your movement with your breath's pace. As you continue to practice yoga in this way, you will find that your breathing naturally becomes deeper, longer, and steadier.

Each time you practice, find the slowest breathing pace you can comfortably sustain. Some days it will be shorter, some days longer. After a stressful day at work, you may find that your breathing pace is faster. On a relaxing Sunday morning, you may find that you can take longer to breathe comfortably and slowly. Many things in your life affect your body, breath, and mind. It is all fine. In yoga, always start with where you are. Become familiar with your breath. It can teach you a lot about yourself.

Principles of Integration:

INHALE to expand.

EXHALE to contract.

Breathing and movement combine in a simple, logical way. Whenever a movement expands your chest or abdomen, you inhale. Conversely, when a movement compresses your chest or abdomen, you exhale.

1. Bending forward contracts your torso, so you exhale. As you come up, you are expanding, so you inhale.

CONTRACT:
EXHALE

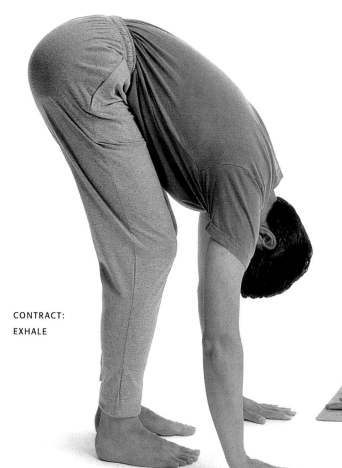

2. You inhale when you arch your back because arching opens up your torso. You exhale when you come back to a neutral position.

ARCH:
INHALE

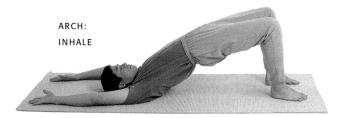

3. Twisting pushes the air out of your lungs in much the same way as you wring water out from a wet dishrag. So you exhale as you twist, and then inhale as you untwist.

TWIST:
EXHALE

4. When you move your legs and arms out from your body, it opens and expands, so you inhale. You exhale when you bring legs and arms back in, compressing your torso.

ARMS AND LEGS MOVE
AWAY FROM BODY:
INHALE

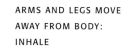

These are the basic breathing and movement principles for all yoga poses. They will come naturally after you've been practicing yoga for a while.

the 2lesson

2.1 ARM RAISE (1.1)

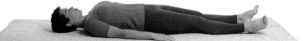

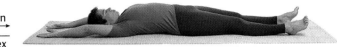

in →
ex ←

Exhaling, lower your arms.

Inhaling, raise your arms.

2.2 STANDING FORWARD BEND (1.4)

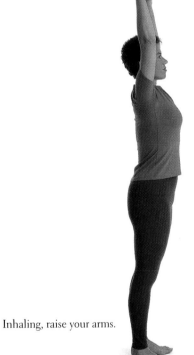

We suggest that you do 4-8 repetitions of each pose, unless otherwise instructed. Over time you will discover how many repetitions benefit you most.

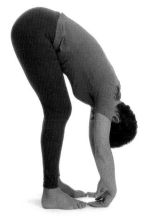

ex →
in ←

Inhaling, raise your arms.

Exhaling, bend forward.

Adapting the Standing Forward Bend

If you are quite stiff or have a back problem that makes forward bends uncomfortable, you can adapt the Forward Bend in several ways:

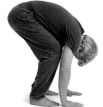

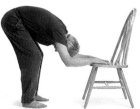

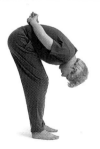

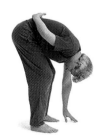

Bend your knees more.

Place your hands on a bench or chair when you bend down.

Rest both arms on your back as you bend forward and come up.

Bring one arm to the floor or a chair and rest the other on your back.

1. Stand, with your feet parallel about 2-1/2 to 3-1/2 feet apart.

2. Inhaling, raise your arms from your sides to shoulder level. Keep your elbows slightly bent and your shoulders relaxed. Pause.

3. Exhaling, turn and place your right hand near your left foot, ankle, or calf—whatever feels most comfortable. Bend your left knee. Rest your left hand on your left hip. Pause.

. Inhaling, come up. Pause.

. Repeat. Exhaling, go to the other side.

    4-5x per side, alternating sides.

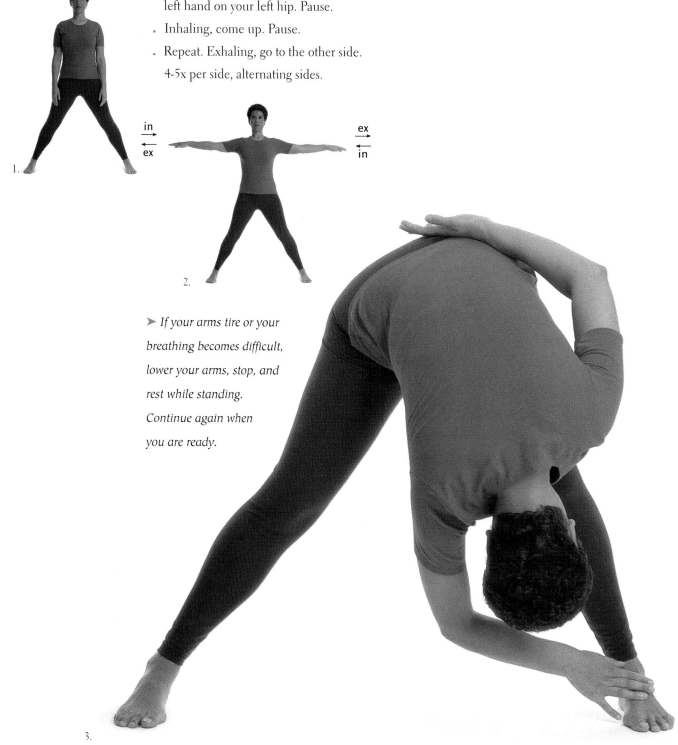

1.

2.

3.

➤ *If your arms tire or your breathing becomes difficult, lower your arms, stop, and rest while standing. Continue again when you are ready.*

- Stand. Place your feet parallel, 6 to 12 inches apart.

1. Inhaling, raise your arms from the front.

2. Exhaling, bend forward with your knees slightly bent. Keep your shoulders and arms relaxed.

3. Take one breath. Inhaling, bend your knees more, allowing your chest and head to raise.

2. Exhaling, straighten your legs somewhat (but never completely! No locked knees!) and stretch down further, with your neck relaxed.

1. Inhaling, come up with your knees slightly bent. Lead with your chest, and keep your arms relaxed.
5-6x

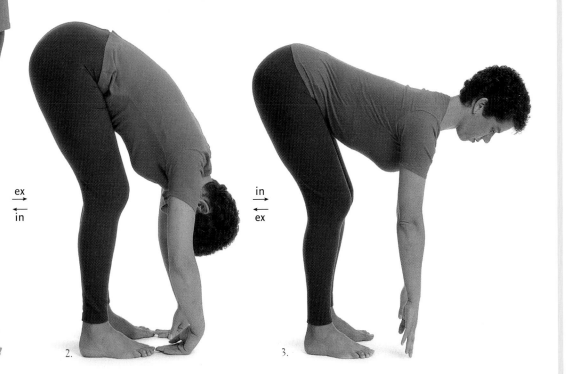

Walk in place or about the room a bit. Then go on to the next pose.

1. Stand. Place your feet parallel, 2 to 3 feet apart.

2. Inhaling, raise your arms from the side to shoulder level.

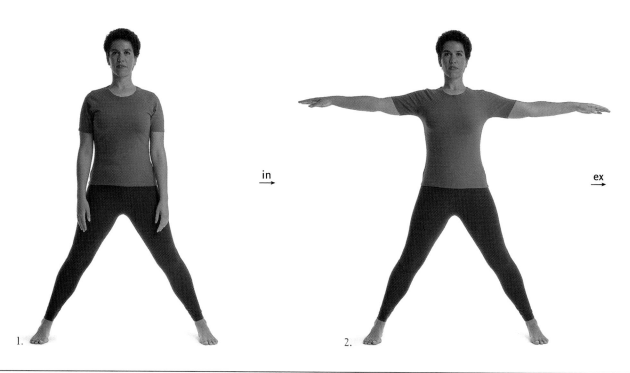

in →

ex →

1.

2.

5. Exhaling, bring your right arm up and out from your right shoulder.

6. Inhaling, come up.

3, 4, 5. Exhaling, bend to the other side. Take one breath, reaching now to the right with your left arm.

6. Inhaling, come up.

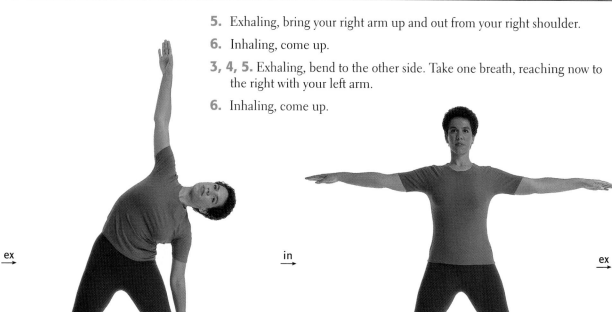

ex →

in →

ex →

5.

6.

3. Exhaling, guide your left hand down your left leg. Grasp your leg firmly just below your bent knee. Relax your head and right arm.

4. Inhaling, reach to the left with your right arm.

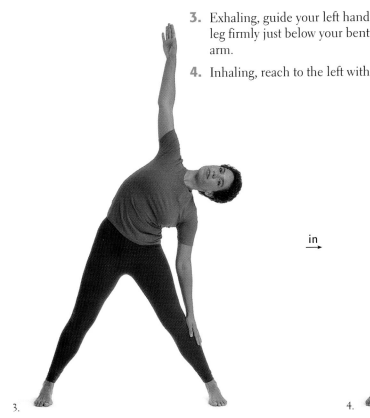

3.

in
→

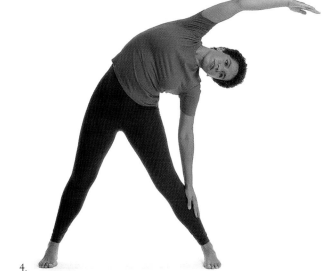

4.

---

7. Exhaling, go into a Forward Bend. Take one breath as you hold the position.

8. Inhaling, come up raising your arms from the side. Relax your arms at shoulder level.

● Continue using this left, right, center combination 3-4 more times.

in
→

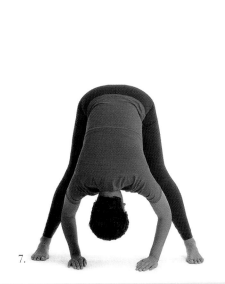

7.

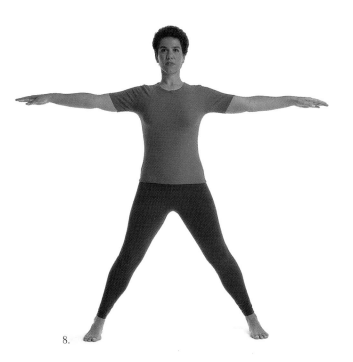

8.

- Lie with your left foot flat on the floor, right leg straight out on the floor. Place your arms at your sides, palms down.

1. Inhaling, raise your arms to the floor over your head. Pause.

2. Exhaling, slowly raise your right leg and lower your arms to your sides. Pause.

1. Inhaling, raise your arms overhead and lower your right leg back to the floor. Pause.

5-6x. Then switch legs.

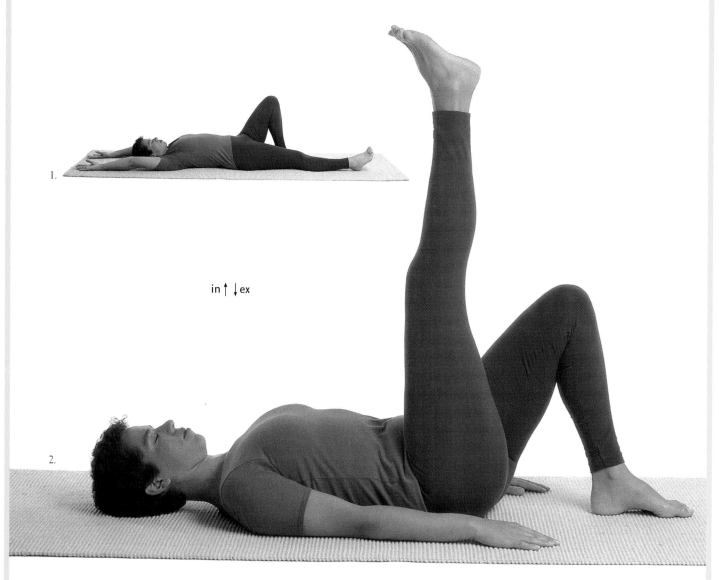

in ↑ ↓ ex

1.

2.

➤ *If you feel tension in your neck or eyes, you may want to place a small pillow under your head and neck.*

Rest briefly. Then go to the next pose.

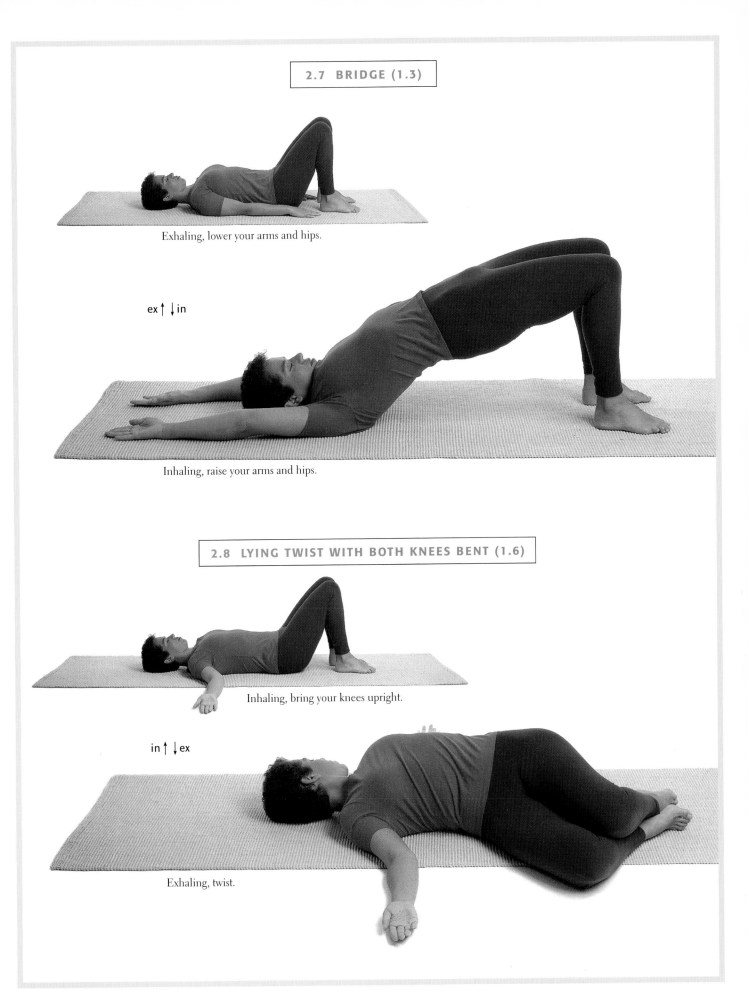

Exhaling, lower your arms and hips.

ex ↑ ↓ in

Inhaling, raise your arms and hips.

2.8 LYING TWIST WITH BOTH KNEES BENT (1.6)

Inhaling, bring your knees upright.

in ↑ ↓ ex

Exhaling, twist.

1. Lie on your back with knees in toward your chest and slightly apart, hands comfortably holding your knees.

2. Inhaling, stretch your legs up and bring your arms to the floor behind you.

1. Exhaling, guide your knees back toward you.

5-6x

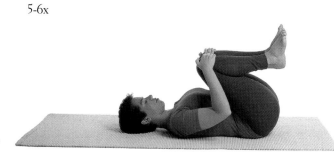

1.

in
$\longrightarrow$
$\longleftarrow$
ex

➤ *If this pose is too difficult, place a small cushion under your head and/or hips. Or practice Upward Leg and Outward Arms Stretch (1.2) instead.*

2.

1. Kneel upright, with your knees slightly apart.

2. Inhaling, raise your arms from the front.

3. Exhaling, bend forward, move your hips back toward your feet and place your hands on the floor.

2. Inhaling, raise your arms and come up to the upright kneeling position.

• Exhaling, lower your arms **(1)**, or bend forward again **(3)**.

5-6x

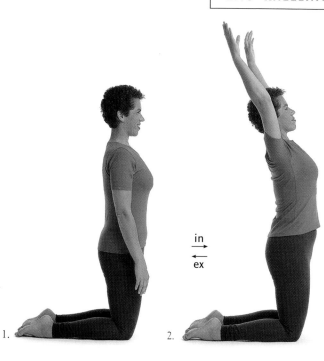

1.

in
$\longrightarrow$
$\longleftarrow$
ex

2.

ex
$\longrightarrow$
$\longleftarrow$
in

3.

➤ *If you lose your balance when coming up, you can bend your arms more or come up using only one arm. If this pose bothers your knees, place small pillows under them. If that doesn't work, skip the pose entirely.*

- Lie in a comfortable resting position. Place your hands on your abdomen or hips, with your shoulders relaxed.

- Inhale comfortably for 3-6 seconds.

- Pause.

- Exhale for a few seconds longer than you inhale.

- Pause.

  Continue for 10-20 breaths.

➤ *Use an easy, comfortable inhalation. With the longer exhalation, bring your attention down toward your abdomen. Relax your face and your eyes. Go more and more deeply inward with each breath.*

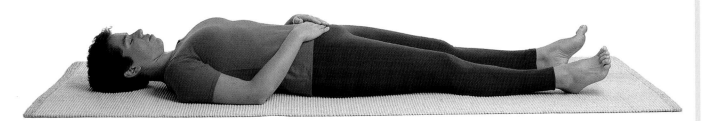

Quietly bring your arms to your sides and rest for 2 minutes.
Take your time to get up and re-enter your day.

Before you progress to the next lesson, remember to practice each lesson until you feel you have mastered the poses and increased your strength and flexibility.

working, relaxing,

working, relaxing,

CONCEPTS & PRINCIPLES

During the weekend you may like to relax by working in your garden. Similarly when you do yoga, you relax by working in the poses. While gardening, you rest your mind by paying attention to the feeling of the soil and the sight of new life pushing up out of it. In yoga, you let go of stress by watching what happens in your breath and movements. The yoga way of relaxing involves working in a focused way—just as gardening does.

Working Your Back in the Best Way

It is important that you bend your knees and relax your elbows while working in poses like the Standing Forward Bend (1.4), The Standing Side Stretch (2.5), and the Triangle Twist to Side (3.3).

Bending your knees in these poses allows your lower back to move more freely, and bending your elbows releases your shoulders and upper back. These adjustments will make you more comfortable and relaxed and will help you avoid injury. They will also allow you to move your back in a way that strengthens it more.

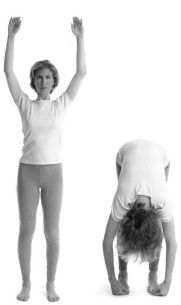

FORWARD BEND (1.4)

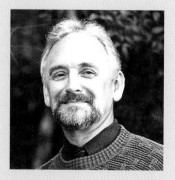

A PHYSICIAN RELIEVES THE ANXIETY OF PUBLIC SPEAKING WITH YOGA

Richard Keenlyside, 51, is an epidemiologist working for the government: "I give many public talks as part of my job. I used to suffer from anxiety and tension in my shoulders before every talk. One time I had to give a speech to 500 people on environmental health. I was very anxious about it. I had to drive for two hours to get there. So before I left, I decided to do my yoga exercises. Then during the drive I continued the yoga breathing. As I focused on long exhalations, my shoulders and hands on the wheel relaxed. When I arrived I was calm and clear-headed. The talk was a breeze!"

and observing

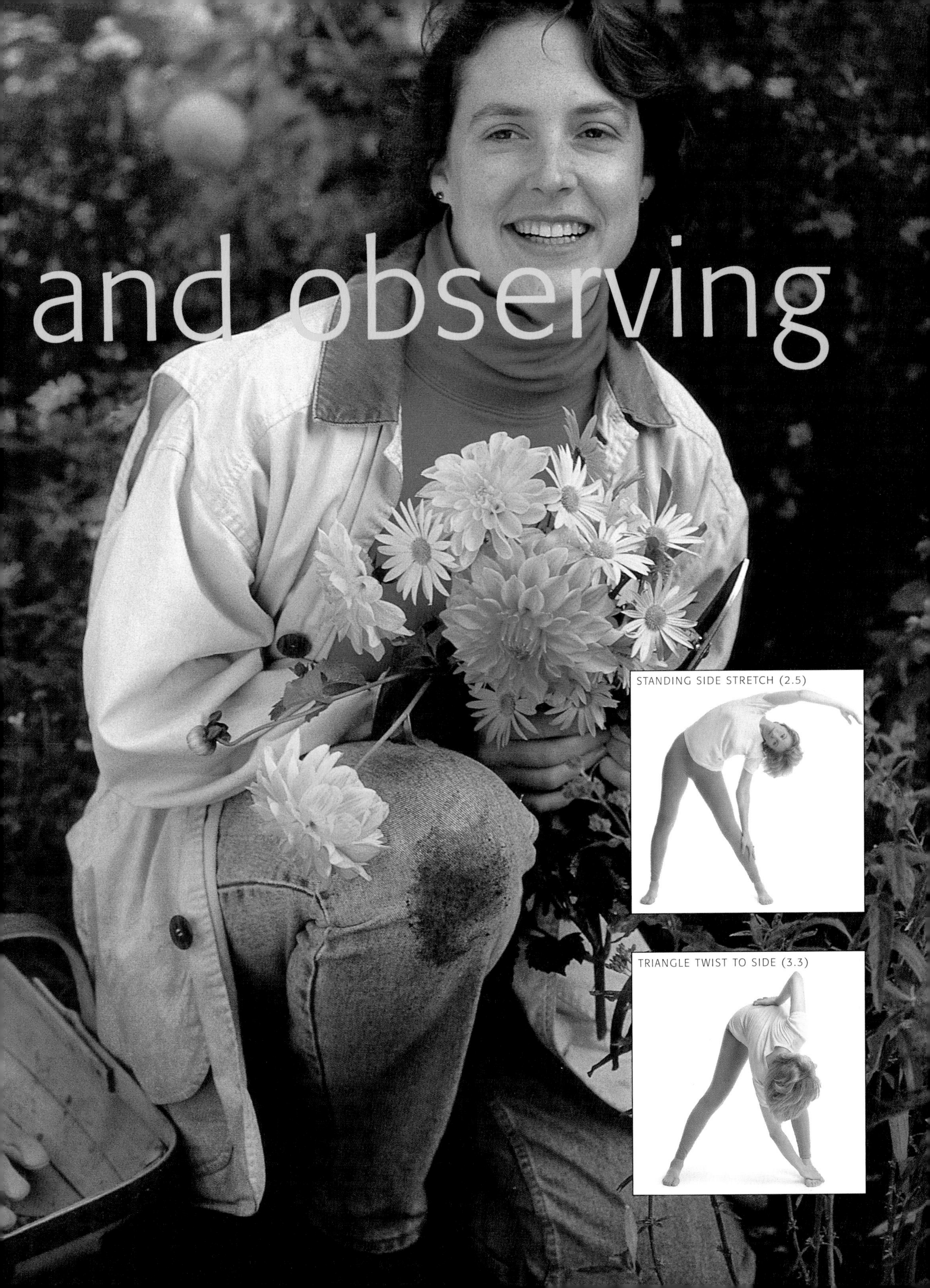

STANDING SIDE STRETCH (2.5)

TRIANGLE TWIST TO SIDE (3.3)

Relaxing Your Neck and Eyes

Because so many people suffer from neck and eye tension, we have included the Seated Head Movements (3.11) at the end of this lesson. You can practice these simple head-tipping and turning movements anytime—in a chair at your desk or as a passenger in a car. You might even sneak them into a boring meeting. You can practice these movements on their own; you don't have to prepare for them with all the other poses in this lesson, although they might be more effective if you did.

The Head Movements may provide you with a quick fix when your neck feels uncomfortable, but they won't prevent the tension from coming back. To do that, you probably need to loosen and relax your neck, shoulders, and back with regular yoga practice. And, of course, it is important to practice good sitting, standing, and sleeping posture.

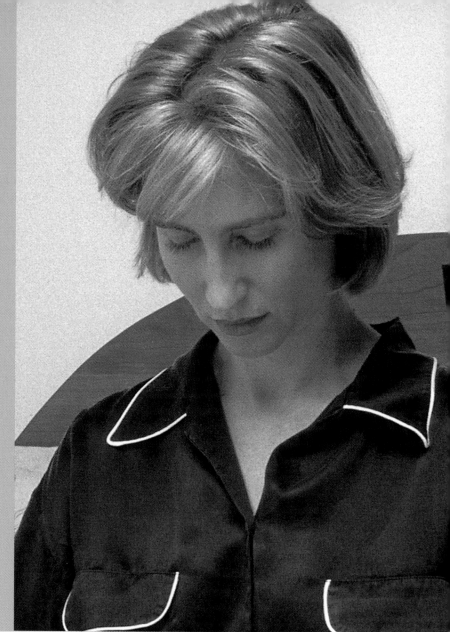

Observing Yourself

Yoga helps you observe your body and spirit. It releases your intuition so that you can better understand the poses and activities that bring you into a better mental and spiritual state. To help you develop the habit of self-observation, use the Visualization Raising One Arm (3.12). As you practice it, ask such questions as: "Am I inclined to practice more with one side of my body than the other? Can I breathe more easily on one side? Can I relax more on one side?" Over time, you can bring this self-awareness to all of the poses that you practice.

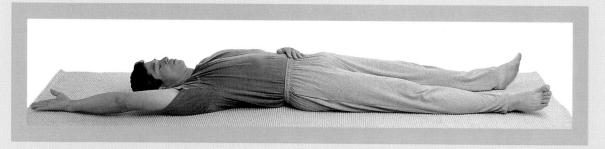

the lesson 3

3.1 ARM RAISE WITH PELVIC TILT

- Lie on your back. Place your feet flat on the floor, hip-distance apart. Place your arms alongside you, palms down.
- Inhaling, raise your arms over your head to the floor.
- Exhaling, lower your arms.

  4-5x

Now that you've loosened up, add a Pelvic Tilt.

- Inhaling, raise your arms over your head to the floor.

1. Exhaling, lower your arms and tilt your pelvis up toward you, flattening your lower back gently to the floor.

2. Inhaling, raise your arms and tilt your pelvis away from you, allowing your knees to come slightly apart. Arch your back slightly, allowing it to rise a little off the floor.

  4-5x

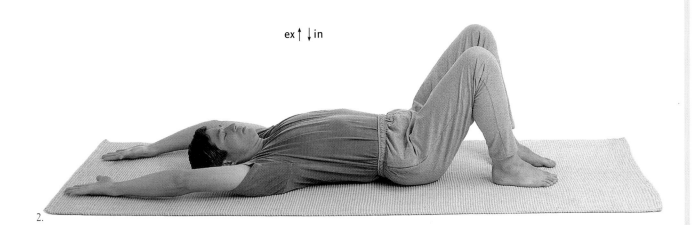

1.

ex ↑ ↓ in

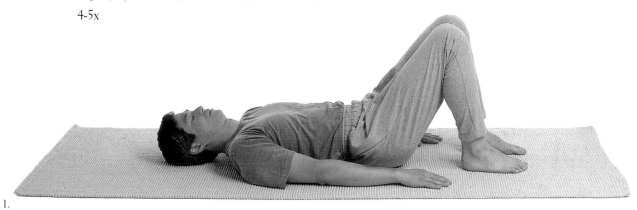

2.

3.2 STANDING FORWARD BEND (1.4)

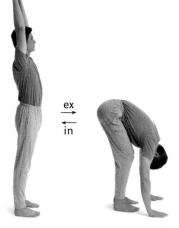

ex →
← in

Inhaling, raise your arms.   Exhaling, bend forward.

3.3 TRIANGLE TWIST TO SIDE

- Stand. Place your feet parallel, about 2-1/2 to 3-1/2 feet apart.

1. Inhaling, raise your arms from the sides to shoulder level.

2. Exhaling, turn toward the left, placing your right hand near your left foot or ankle. Bend your left knee. Turn your left shoulder gently back as you twist your torso.

- Take one breath, inhaling in place **(2)**. Exhaling, twist your torso a bit more if you can.

1. Inhaling, come up.

2. Exhaling, twist to the other side.

4-5x per side, alternating sides.

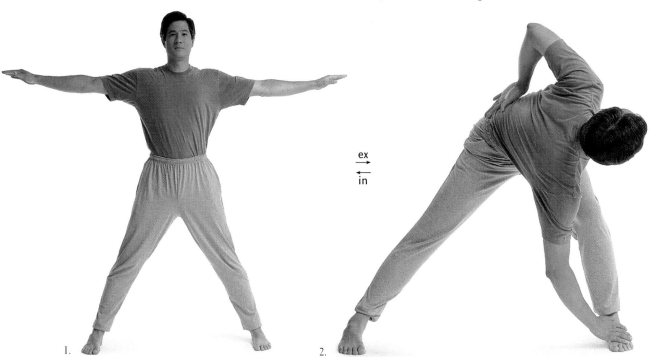

ex →
← in

1.   2.

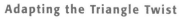

Adapting the Triangle Twist

If you have back problems or if you are stiff, you may put your hand on a low bench for the Triangle Twist to Side (3.3). Although the picture to the right shows one bench, you may want to place a bench by each foot.

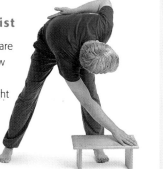

3.4 STANDING FORWARD BEND WITH LEG STRETCH (2.4)

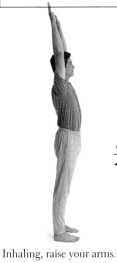 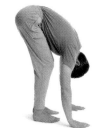 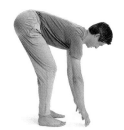

Inhaling, raise your arms.   Exhaling, bend forward.   Inhaling, arch your back.

3.5 STANDING SIDE STRETCH/FORWARD BEND COMBINATION (2.5)

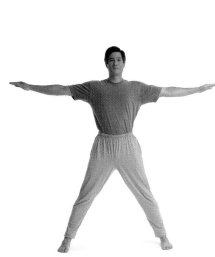 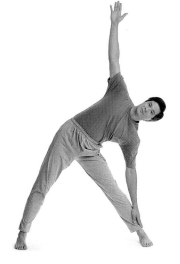 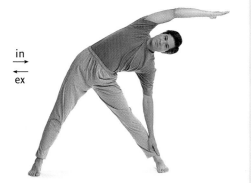

Inhaling, raise your arms.   Exhaling, bend to the side.   Inhaling, extend your arm.

Practice to the Left and Right

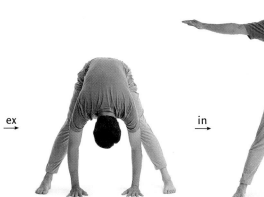 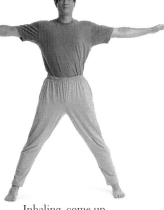

Exhaling, bend forward.   Inhaling, come up.

3.6 LEG LIFT, LOWERING FOOT ALMOST TO THE FLOOR

1. Lie with your left foot flat on the floor, and your right leg straight out on the floor. Place your arms at your sides, palms down.

● Inhaling, raise your arms to the floor over your head.

2. Exhaling, raise your right leg slowly and lower your arms to your sides.

3. Inhaling, raise your arms overhead and lower your right leg bringing your right heel about 1 inch from the floor.

2. Exhaling, lower your arms and raise your right leg again.

5-6x, then practice with your left leg.

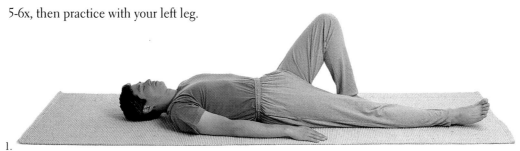

1.

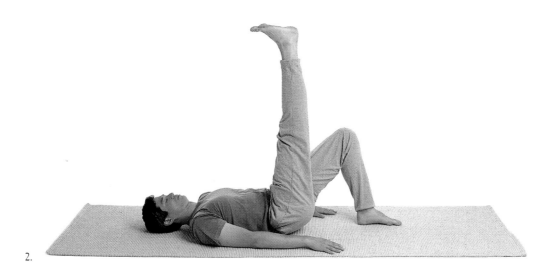

2.

ex ↑ ↓ in

Lower foot to about 1 inch off the floor.

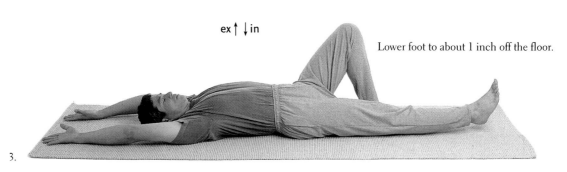

3.

➤ *If this variation is too difficult go back to the easier Leg Lift (2.6).*

Rest briefly before going on.

3.7 BRIDGE (1.3)

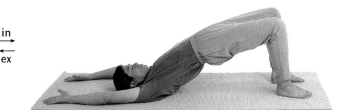

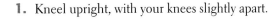

Exhaling, lower your arms and hips.

Inhaling, raise your arms and hips.

3.8 KNEELING FORWARD BEND/CAT

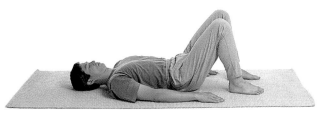

1. Kneel upright, with your knees slightly apart.

2. Inhaling, raise your arms from the front.

3. Exhaling, bend forward, moving your hips back to your feet and placing your hands on the floor.

4. Inhaling, move forward arching your back gently and raising your head slightly.

3. Exhaling, move back again.

2. Inhaling, come up to the upright kneeling position.

1. Exhaling, lower your arms.

   5-6x.

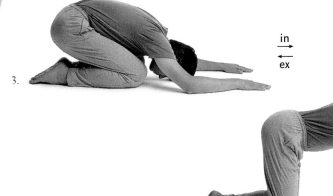

➤ *If it bothers you to kneel, try the Cat (1.7) instead.*

3.9 LYING TWIST WITH ONE KNEE BENT

1. Lie with your left foot on the floor near your right knee. Spread your arms out to your sides, palms up.

2. Exhaling, bring your left knee to the right near the floor. Rest your left foot on the inside of your right knee.

1. Inhaling, bring your knee back to the original position **(1)**. Repeat.

2. If you feel comfortable in the twist position, exhale and hold the twist for one breath.

• Inhaling, keep your left knee down to the floor on the right side.

• Exhaling, bring your left knee further to the right and gently press your left shoulder down toward the floor.

1. Inhaling, return to your original position **(1)**.

3-5x per side.

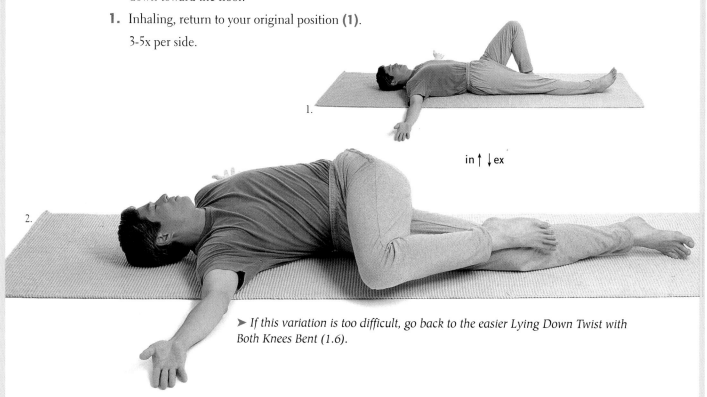

in ↑ ↓ex

➤ *If this variation is too difficult, go back to the easier Lying Down Twist with Both Knees Bent (1.6).*

Adapting the Lying Twist

If your shoulders bother you in either of the Lying Twists (1.6 or 3.9), you may place your hands so that they slide comfortably on your abdomen or chest.

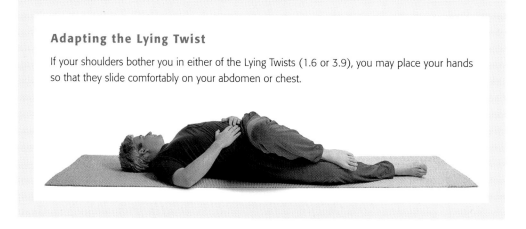

3.10 UPWARD LEGS AND ARMS STRETCH (2.9)

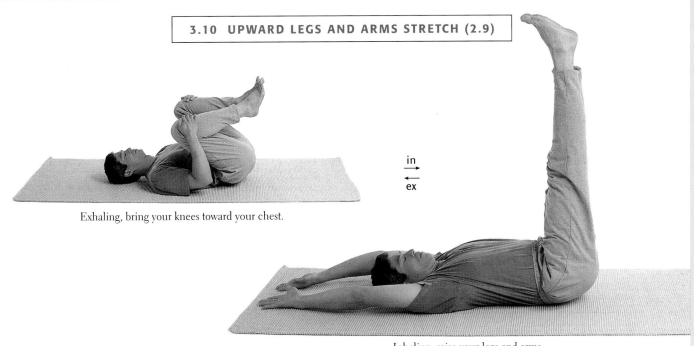

Exhaling, bring your knees toward your chest.

in
ex

Inhaling, raise your legs and arms.

3.11 SEATED HEAD MOVEMENTS

- Sit comfortably on a chair with your feet flat on the floor, shoulders relaxed, and hands comfortably settled on your thighs.

1. Inhaling, gently tilt your head back.

2. Exhaling, lower your head slowly down. Relax your facial muscles and eyes.

   2-4x

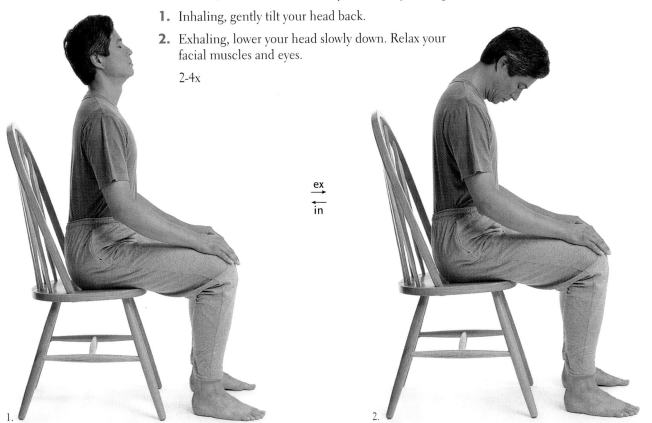

ex
in

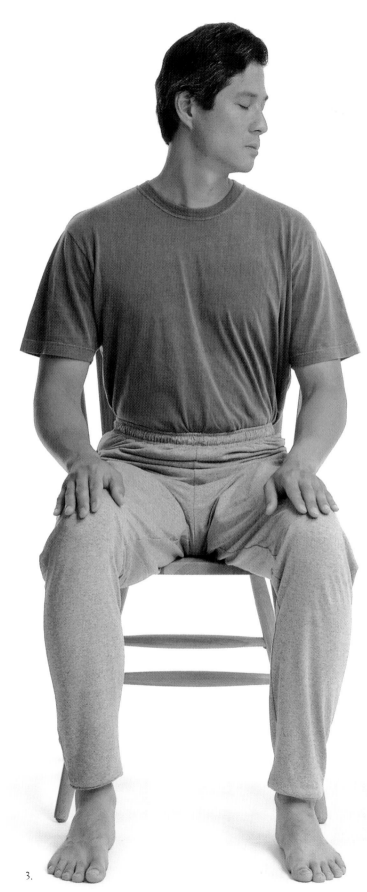

- Inhaling, raise your head so that it faces straight ahead.

3. Exhaling, turn your head to one side.

- Inhaling, bring your head to the front.

- Exhaling, turn your head to the other side.

- Inhaling, bring your head to the front.

  2-3x per side, alternating sides.

  Conclude by moving your head forward and back **(1 & 2)**.

  2-3x

➤ *People tend to overdo Head Movements. To avoid over-stretching, keep your shoulders relaxed and move your head gently in the four directions.*

3.

1. Lie in the rest position. Place your left hand on your left hip and your right arm alongside you, palm down.

2. Inhaling, breathe into the right side of your chest as you raise your right arm overhead. Visualize bringing a relaxing energy into the right side of your body. Pause a few seconds.

1. Exhaling, lower your right arm and relax the right side of your body. Think of letting go through your entire right side—forehead, eye, face, chest, arm, leg, hand, foot, fingers, and toes. Pause a few seconds.

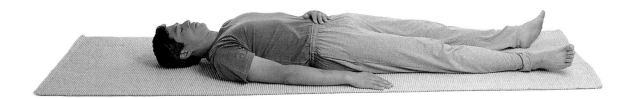

ex ↑ ↓ in

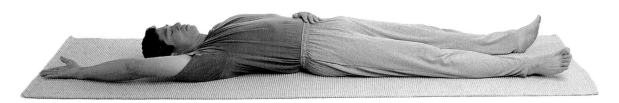

- Bring your attention more and more deeply inward, relaxing with each breath.

   5-6x with your right arm, then 5-6x with your left arm.

   Then try raising both arms together 1-2x.

Rest for two minutes with your arms by your sides or place your hands on your hips or abdomen.

the art of sequencing

CONCEPTS & PRINCIPLES

The Sequence of Poses

There is a logic to the sequence of poses in this yoga tradition. You may have already noticed this in the first three lessons. The sequencing of poses is an art.

Poses can be arranged in many different ways to produce a variety of effects on your body, breath, and mind. By choosing the right poses and the right sequence, a trained teacher can develop a program that addresses the individual's specific needs.

In this book, the flow of poses is designed to give you an overall feeling of energy, relaxation, and focus. However, if you don't have time to do all the poses in a given lesson, you can stop before the end of the program. If you stop before you finish the lesson, please make sure that your last pose does not need a counterpose. (We will explain what a counterpose is shortly.) Or, if you do a few poses from a lesson and then stop for a few hours, please don't try to pick up where you left off. You will be safer if you start again right from the beginning of the lesson.

The photographs on the next few pages demonstrate the basic principles involved in sequencing a yoga program: warming up, working a little harder, relaxing, and counterposes. **(These pictures are for illustration only; please don't try these poses now.)**

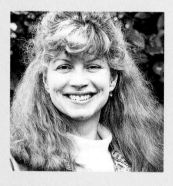

A SPEECH THERAPIST USES YOGA TO HELP STUTTERERS

Kim Papastavridis is a 39-year-old speech pathologist: "I use the yoga that I have learned from the Pierces to help stutterers and people with speech problems. The slow and focused breathing helps them become more relaxed and less nervous. Their therapy is more effective. Also, they can do the yoga breathing very unobtrusively on their own, in public, at work, or wherever."

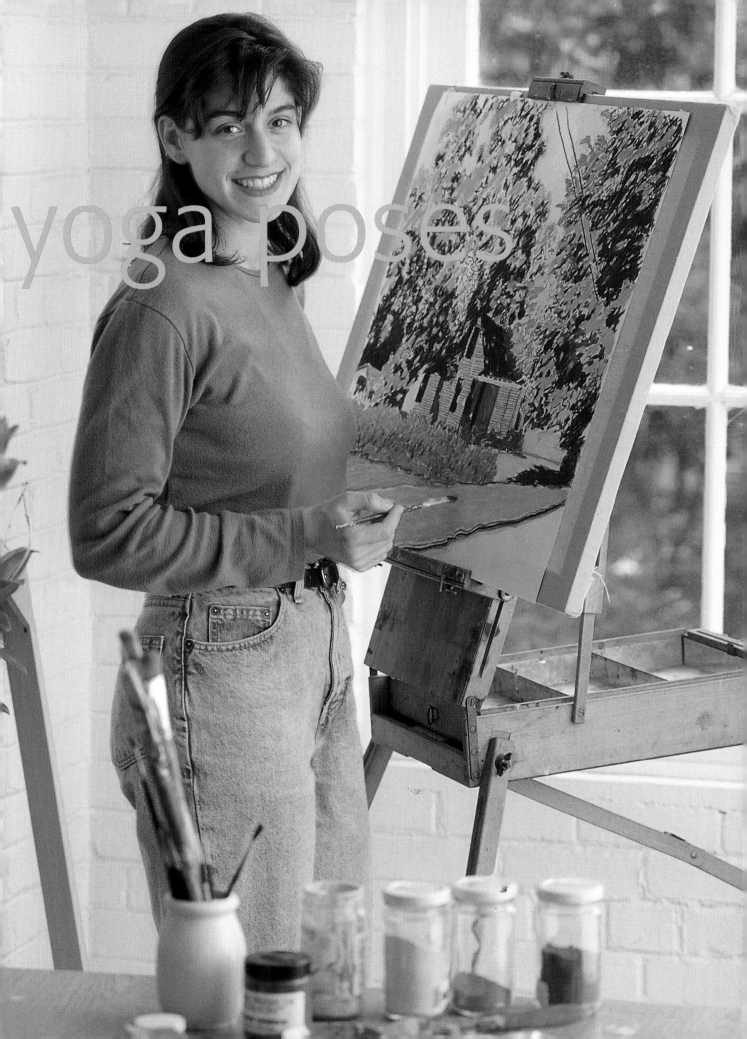

yoga poses

Warm Up First

Many lessons begin with gentle and uncomplicated poses to warm your muscles and help you become more aware of your body—especially your breathing. For instance, Lesson 4 starts with the simple Tree pose (4.1).

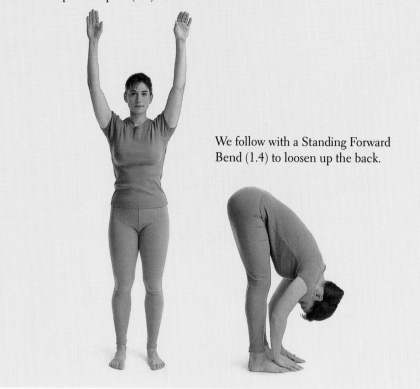

We follow with a Standing Forward Bend (1.4) to loosen up the back.

Then Work a Little Harder:

Then we introduce more demanding standing poses, such as the Standing Head to Knee Pose (4.3) and the Triangle Twist to Center (4.4).

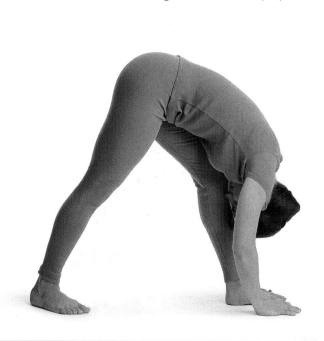

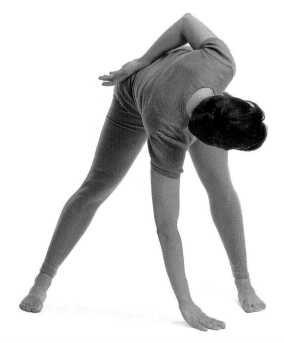

Then we ask you to practice some easy kneeling or lying poses, such as the Bridge (1.3). These are intended to relax you and help you focus on your breath after the strenuous movements.

We progress to the more difficult Cobra (4.9) and Locust (4.10) poses, while lying on your stomach.

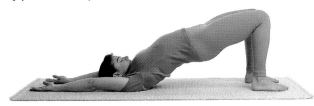

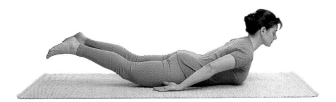

We follow these with milder poses like Kneeling Forward Bend, Sweeping Arms (4.12).

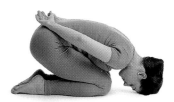

Relax at the End

Having energized and relaxed your body, and cleared the cobwebs out of your mind, you can focus your attention on a breathing pose, such as the wonderfully relaxing Lying Visualization, Raising One Arm (3.12). Or, depending on your mood, you can lie down and gradually extend your hold out after exhalation as we present in 4.14, or you can do a simple neck and eye relaxer like the Seated Head Movements (3.11).

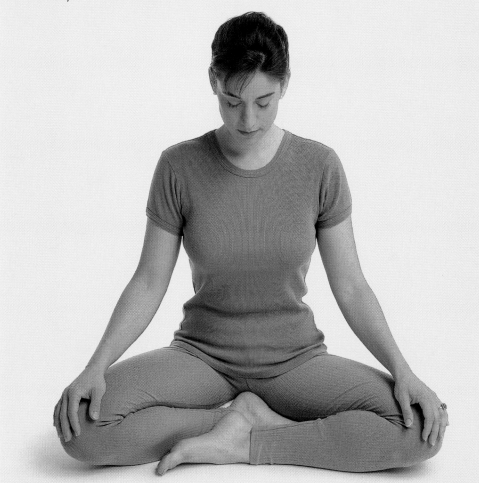

Counterposes

Counterposes help bring your body into balance after a strong pose or movement. If you don't follow some strong poses with a counterpose, you might strain or injure yourself. For instance, after doing a Triangle Twist to Side (3.3) or a Standing Side Stretch (2.5) you need to straighten out your spine with a Standing Forward Bend variation (2.4) or (4.5).

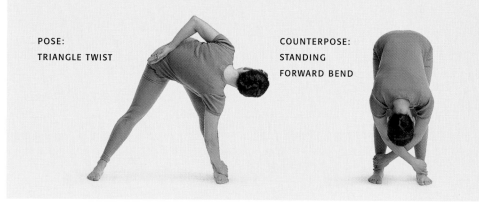

POSE:
TRIANGLE TWIST

COUNTERPOSE:
STANDING
FORWARD BEND

After a lying twist variation (1.6) or (3.9), you may do the Knees to Chest Pose (1.5) or the Upward Legs and Arms Stretch (2.9).

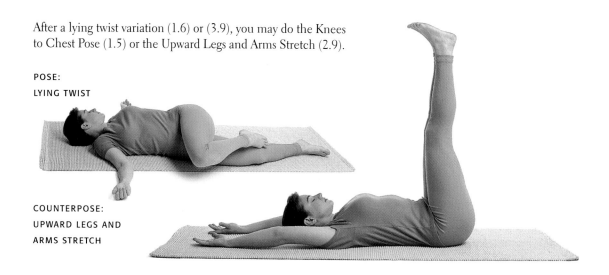

POSE:
LYING TWIST

COUNTERPOSE:
UPWARD LEGS AND
ARMS STRETCH

If a pose pushes you strongly in one direction, you may need a counterpose that moves you gently in the opposite direction. For instance, the Cobra (4.9) and Locust (4.10) arch your back strongly. These poses are powerful back strengtheners. They may help you to stand straighter and avoid back problems.

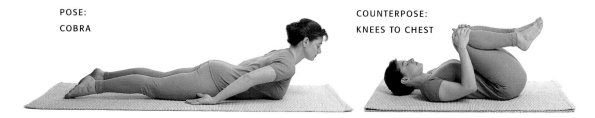

POSE:
COBRA

COUNTERPOSE:
KNEES TO CHEST

After practicing poses that arch your back strongly, you need to follow with something that gently flattens your back, such as the Knees to Chest Pose (1.5).

When you use the principles of proper sequencing, you will be able to practice yoga safely with many beneficial effects.

the lesson 4

4.1 TREE

1. Stand with your feet parallel, 6 to 12 inches apart, with your arms at your sides.

2. Inhaling, raise your arms slowly from the front to a comfortable position, elbows bent, hands relaxed. Pause.

1. Exhaling, lower your arms to the side. Pause.

5-6x

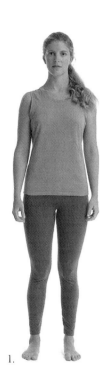 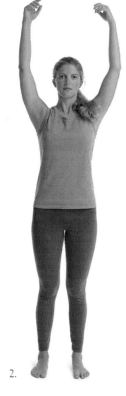

in →
← ex

1.   2.

4.2 STANDING FORWARD BEND (1.2)

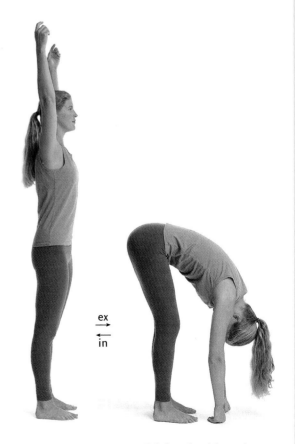

ex →
← in

Inhaling, raise your arms.   Exhaling, bend forward.

1. Stand with your left foot 2 to 3-1/2 feet forward. Turn your right foot out slightly.

2. Inhaling, raise your arms from the front.

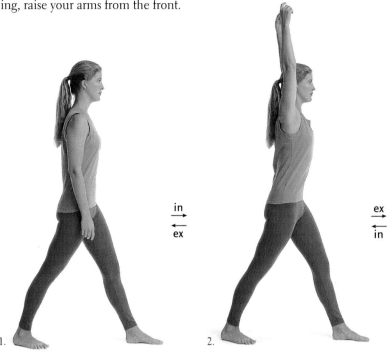

1.   2.

| 4.4 TRIANGLE TWIST TO CENTER |

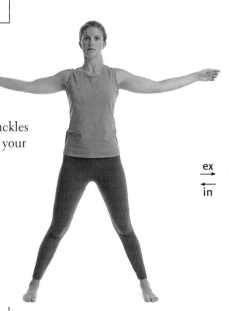

• Stand, feet parallel, 2-1/2 to 3-1/2 feet apart.

1. Inhaling, raise your arms from the sides to shoulder level.

2. Exhaling, turn and place your right hand, fingers, or your knuckles on the floor in front of you, slightly to the left of center. Bend your knees a little. Turn your left shoulder gently back as you twist your torso.

3. Take one breath in the twist, arching your back as you inhale and move your chest forward.

2. As you exhale, twist to the left a bit more.

1. Inhaling, come up to standing.

   4-6x per side, alternating sides.

1.

3. Exhaling, bend forward, bending your left knee slightly and placing your hands to either side of your left foot.

4. Inhaling, slightly raise your chest and head.

3. Exhaling, lower your chest and head.

2. Inhaling, come up leading with your chest and relaxed arms.

4-6x, equally to each side.

➤ *If you are unstable, put your back heel against a wall. If you are tight, try bending forward to a chair or stool.*

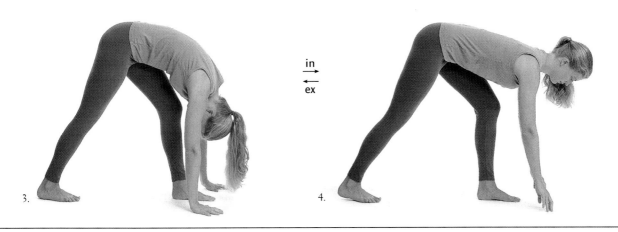

in
⟶
⟵
ex

3.

4.

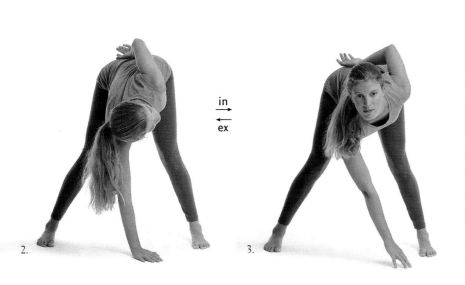

in
⟶
⟵
ex

2.

3.

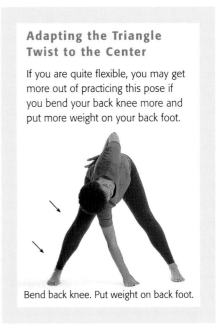

Adapting the Triangle Twist to the Center

If you are quite flexible, you may get more out of practicing this pose if you bend your back knee more and put more weight on your back foot.

Bend back knee. Put weight on back foot.

4.5 STANDING FORWARD BEND, FOREARMS CROSSED

1. Stand, feet parallel, 6 to 12 inches apart.

2. Inhaling, raise your arms from the front.

3. Exhaling, bend forward, lower your arms from the side, cross your forearms, and lightly grasp the outside of your feet, ankles, or calves.

• Take one breath.

2. Inhaling, extend your arms and come up leading with your chest and arms relaxed. Pause.

• Exhaling, continue bending forward (3), or lower your arms (1).

4-6x

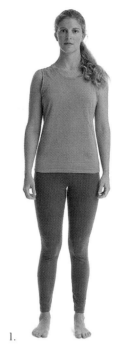

in
ex

1.

4.6 KNEELING FORWARD BEND/UP-FACE DOG SEQUENCE

1. Kneel upright, with your knees slightly apart and arms by your sides.

2. Inhaling, raise your arms from the front.

3. Exhaling, bend forward, moving your hips back towards your feet and placing your hands and elbows on the floor.

4. Inhaling, move forward into the Up-Face Dog, arching your back and keeping your knees *on* the floor.

3. Exhaling, return to the hips back position.

2. Inhaling, come up to an upright kneeling position.

1. Exhaling, lower your arms.

4-6x

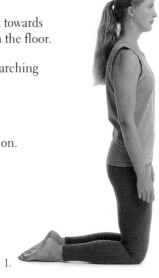

in
ex

1.

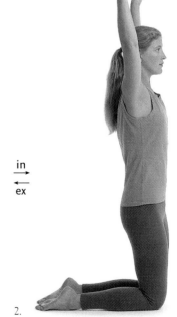

ex
in

2.

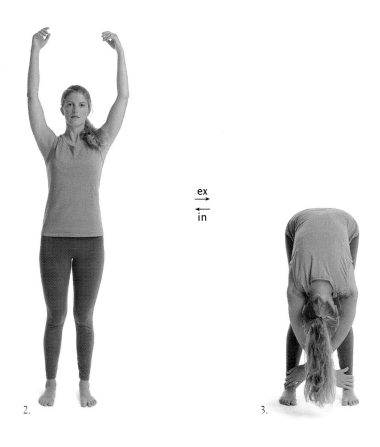

$$\xrightarrow{\text{ex}}$$
$$\xleftarrow{\text{in}}$$

2.

3.

➤ *If the Up-Face Dog bothers your wrists, back, or shoulders, try moving only part way forward as you inhale, or use the Cat arch instead. If you want to work harder, you can move back and forth between the Kneeling Forward Bend and the Up-Face Dog two or three times before coming into the upright kneeling position.*

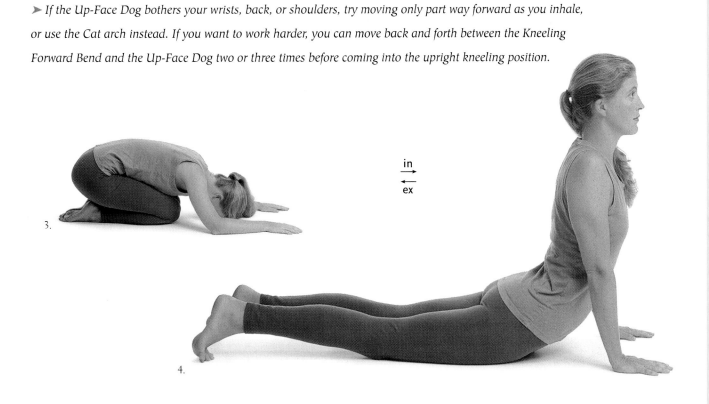

3.

$$\xrightarrow{\text{in}}$$
$$\xleftarrow{\text{ex}}$$

4.

4.7 UPWARD LEGS AND ARMS STRETCH (2.9)

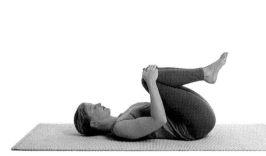

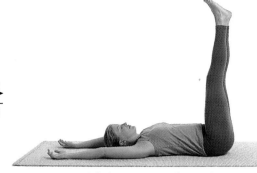

in →

ex ←

Exhaling, bring your knees toward your chest.

Inhaling, raise your legs and arms.

4.8 BRIDGE (1.3)

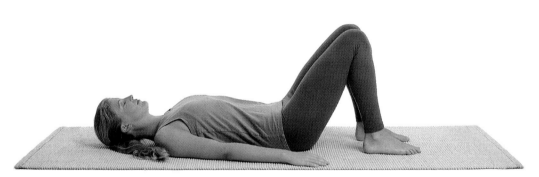

Exhaling, lower your arms and hips.

ex ↑ ↓ in

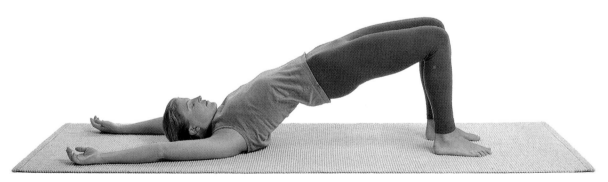

Inhaling, raise your arms and hips.

1. Lie on your stomach, with your forehead on the floor and your legs slightly apart, arms along-side you, palms up.

2. Inhaling, come up, raising your chest, gradually lifting your head slightly back. Pause.

1. Exhaling, relax down to the floor. Pause.

    4-5x.

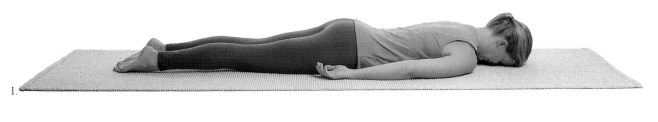

1.

➤ *Be sure that you come up gently and slowly. Don't strain as you come up. Yoga gives no prize for height in the Cobra. If your body is tight, you will work hard even if you come up only a little way. Avoid over working your neck. Instead, come up using your back muscles.*

ex ↑ ↓ in

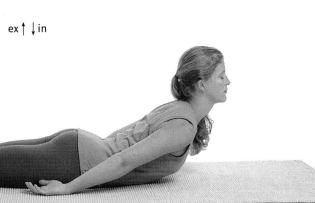

2.

Adapting the Cobra

If this Cobra variation is too difficult, try the following adaptations to strengthen and loosen your back:

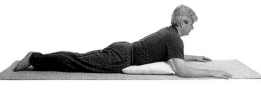

Adaptation 1: Place a soft pillow under your abdomen. Bring your legs further apart and place your arms comfortably on the floor in front of you, elbows out to the side of your shoulders. Inhaling, come up, with your forearms on the floor for gentle support.

Adaptation 2: Inhaling, come all the way up resting your weight on your palms for support. Keep your legs well apart and your navel on the floor. You may choose to use a pillow or not.

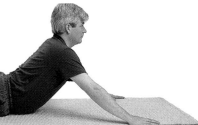

Feel free to experiment with different hand and arm placements to find the most effective position for you.

1. Remain on your stomach.

2. Inhaling, raise your chest and both legs. Pause.

1. Exhaling, come down to the floor. Pause.

4-5x

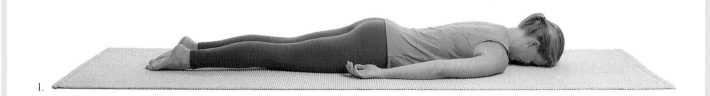

1.

ex ↑ ↓ in

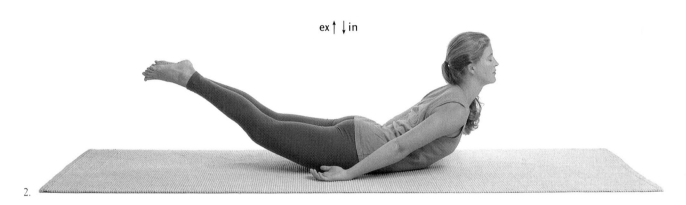

2.

➤ *If the Cobra or the Locust are too difficult, skip them and go on to the next pose.*

4.11 KNEE TO CHEST POSE (1.5)

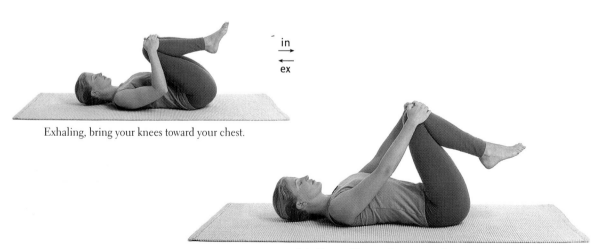

in
→
ex

Exhaling, bring your knees toward your chest.

Inhaling, guide your knees away from you.

4.12 KNEELING FORWARD BEND, SWEEPING ARMS

1. Kneel upright, knees slightly apart.

2. Inhaling, raise your arms from the front.

3. Exhaling, bend forward, sweep your arms behind you and place your hands on your lower back.

2. Inhaling, come up leading with your arms and chest.

• Exhaling, repeat the pose **(3)**, or simply lower your arms to the side **(1)**.

  5-6x

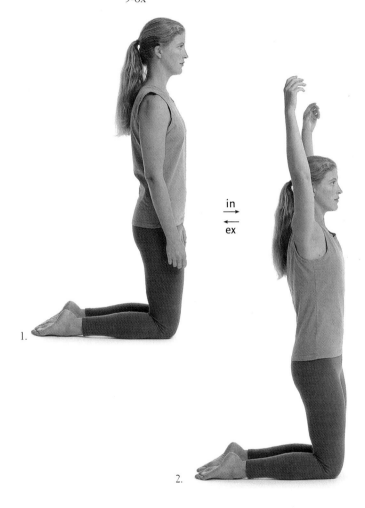

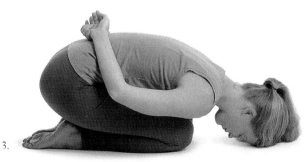

1. Lie on your back with your knees comfortably toward you, one hand near each knee.

2. Inhaling, straighten your legs, with your feet 0 to 12 inches apart. Gently grasp the backs of your knees or thighs.

3. Exhaling, slightly bend your knees.

• Inhaling, straighten your legs again **(2)**. Continue for several breaths. Bend slightly as you exhale **(3)** and straighten as you inhale **(2)**.

1. Finally, bring your knees back toward your chest gently pressing your lower back toward the floor. Repeat.

   2-3x

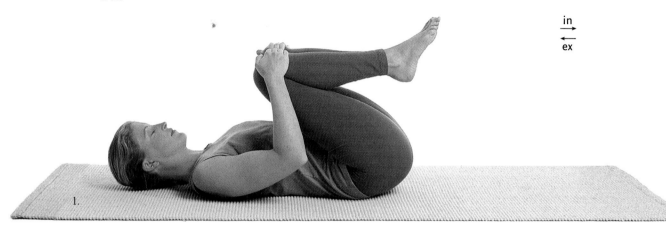

in
→
←
ex

Extending the Hold Out After Exhalation

• Lie comfortably on your back. Place your hands on your lower abdomen and close your eyes.

• Take a few easy breaths to relax your body.

• Continue with easy inhalations and exhalations, and begin to hold your breath out, suspending it after your exhalations for two seconds. Do this 2-3x.

• Every two to three breaths, increase the time you hold your breath out by one second, up to a maximum of six seconds. Keep your attention in your abdominal area as you gently exhale and hold your breath out.

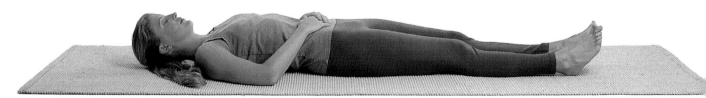

Hold OUT 2, 3, 4, 5, 6 seconds   2-3 breaths each count.

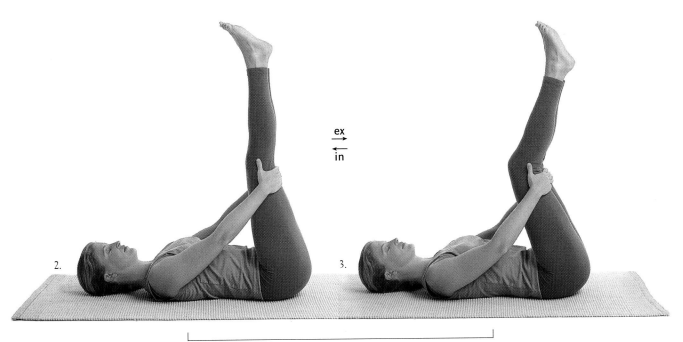

2.

3.

ex →

in ←

Repeat

➤ If this pose makes your legs, back, or neck uncomfortable, pull your knees into your chest with each exhalation. If your head tips back or your hips come up off the floor, place a pillow under them. If you are so flexible that you can place your fingers over your feet, then do so. Notice if it is more comfortable to keep your legs together, 12 inches apart, or even 24 inches apart.

➤ Holding your breath out after exhalation is an important part of yoga breathing. It deepens the release of tensions in your body. It is a time of letting go and stillness. Does it come easily for you? Is a maximum hold out of three seconds your comfortable limit? Or do you feel relaxed with six, seven, or even eight seconds as a maximum hold out? Can you feel a sense of release? Experiment, but remember never to strain.

Rest for 2 minutes.

Work on each lesson for at least a week, maybe two weeks, before moving to the next lesson. Each lesson will help you prepare for the next and will bring you cumulative benefits.

sitting and

The Best Way to Sit

In this lesson we explore seated breathing. For most people, lying down is the easiest and most relaxing position in which to practice breathing. However, sitting in an erect position allows you to be more alert and mentally focused.

A proper seated posture protects your lower back and maintains the normal spinal curve you have when you stand. It allows your rib cage and abdomen to be free of tension and helps you to breathe fully. There is no need to sit fully crossed legged on the floor. In fact, we find that most people must sit up two or more inches on a pillow to achieve the best alignment of their back. This way there is less pressure on your knees, and it is easier to get up when you finish. The important thing is to sit comfortably erect without forcing, so that you can concentrate on your breathing with ease.

Poor posture in itself may produce lower back and neck discomfort or pain. Once back and neck problems develop, poor posture frequently perpetuates the problems and makes them worse. Yoga helps build the strength, flexibility, and awareness to maintain good posture. The following instructions will help you develop stronger and healthier posture.

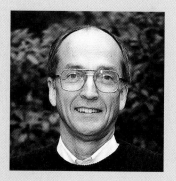

A FINANCIAL OFFICER DOES TWO-MINUTE EXECUTIVE YOGA

Miles Wilson, 58, was chief financial officer of an international engineering company. His schedule took him all over the world with barely any time for relaxation or exercise. He devised what he calls 'Two-Minute Executive Yoga' breaks: "The two-minute yoga breaks quiet my mind. Many thoughts jump at me just after I wake up: plans for the day, things that have to be done, etc. Yoga helps me to focus, to put things into a clear perspective, and to prioritize my time. During the day, the yoga breaks boost my energy to carry me through my meetings. Also yoga helps me relax my back during thirty hour plane trips from Atlanta to Brazil and other places. It makes a big difference in how I feel after I travel."

breathing

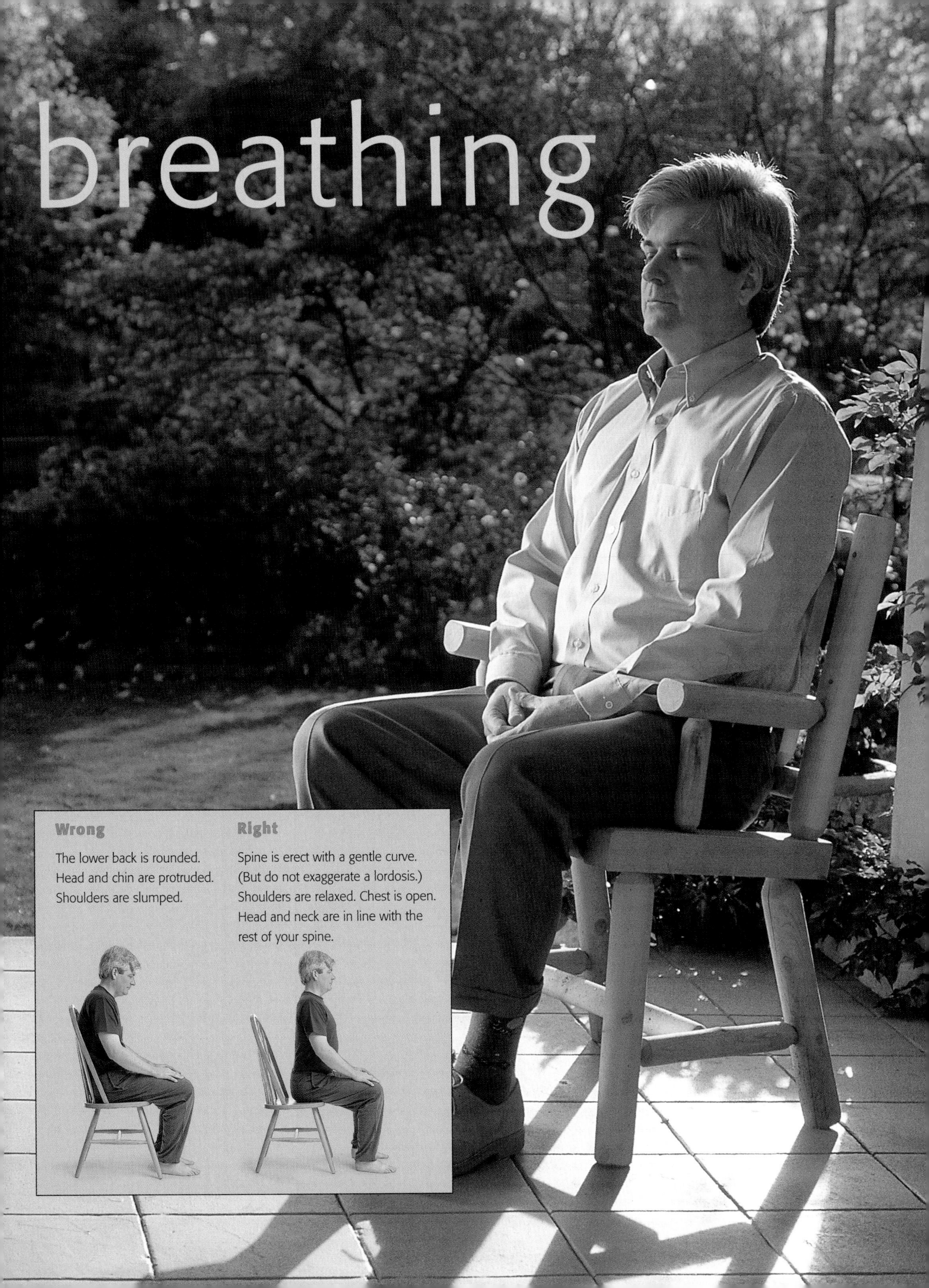

Wrong

The lower back is rounded.
Head and chin are protruded.
Shoulders are slumped.

Right

Spine is erect with a gentle curve.
(But do not exaggerate a lordosis.)
Shoulders are relaxed. Chest is open.
Head and neck are in line with the
rest of your spine.

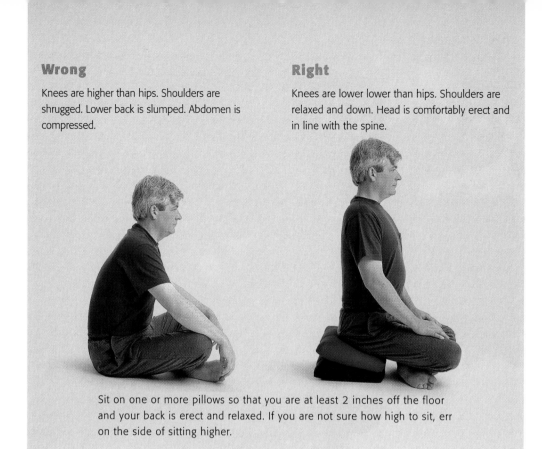

Wrong

Knees are higher than hips. Shoulders are shrugged. Lower back is slumped. Abdomen is compressed.

Right

Knees are lower lower than hips. Shoulders are relaxed and down. Head is comfortably erect and in line with the spine.

Sit on one or more pillows so that you are at least 2 inches off the floor and your back is erect and relaxed. If you are not sure how high to sit, err on the side of sitting higher.

Understanding Inhalation and Exhalation

Your inhalation and exhalation establish a constant flow of energy and release within you. As you learn to balance your energizing inhalation and releasing exhalation, you will begin to balance the qualities of vitality and relaxation in your body and mind. As you practice, your breathing should improve. The following are some guidelines for effective breathing.

Inhalation:

The inhalation brings continuous energy into your body. When you first start practicing yoga, your chest may feel somewhat tight, and it may be easier to inhale by expanding your abdomen. As you continue to practice you will be able to start your inhalation higher up in your chest. Imagine breathing into this spot, which like a balloon expands upwards, sideways, and down into your abdomen. In this way, you will maximize the effectiveness of each inhalation, bringing more oxygen and energy into your system.

If you find that chest inhalation causes you neck or shoulder tension, we urge you to inhale less deeply or go back to abdominal breathing until your torso and intercostal muscles are more stretched and relaxed.

Exhalation:

The exhalation is the most important part of the breath because it heals and relaxes you. Start your exhale by gently contracting your lower abdomen. Then gently contract your upper abdomen and allow the air to flow out of your chest. If you are doing a pose, your exhalation will probably be from 4-10 seconds long. If you are lying still, it may be longer. The length of the breath depends on the posture. Your exhalation should always be as long as or longer than your inhalation.

the 5 lesson

Remember to do at least 4 but usually no more than 8 repetitions of the poses that you have learned in previous lessons. You need at least 4 repetitions to fully work your muscles and bring your attention more deeply inward. More than 8 repetitions may unnecessarily tire you.

5.1 VISUALIZATION RAISING ONE ARM (3.12)

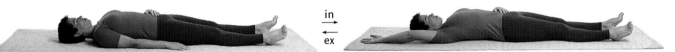

Exhaling, lower your arm.

Inhaling, raise your arm.

5.2 UPWARD LEGS AND OUTWARD ARMS STRETCH

1. Lie on your back with your hands comfortably holding your knees toward your chest.

2. Inhaling, stretch your legs up and bring your arms out to the sides.

1. Exhaling, bring your knees back toward you, hands on your knees, pressing your lower back gently toward the floor.

5-6x

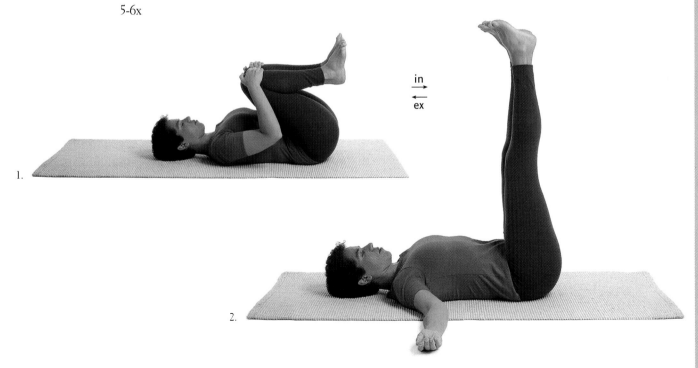

➤ *Bringing your arms to the sides, instead of to the floor over your head, is often easier on your neck and more relaxing, especially if you are tired.*

5.3 BRIDGE (1.3)

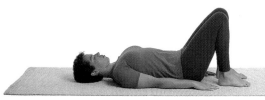

Exhaling, lower your arms and hips.

$$\begin{array}{c}\text{in} \\ \longrightarrow \\ \longleftarrow \\ \text{ex}\end{array}$$

Inhaling, raise your arms and hips.

5.4a STANDING FORWARD BEND, SWEEPING ARMS

AND 5.4b COMING UP PART WAY

- Stand with your feet parallel and 6 to 12 inches apart.

1. Inhaling, raise your arms from the front.

2. Exhaling, bend forward lowering your arms from the side. Rest your hands on your lower back, palms out. Just pause, or pause and take one breath.

1. Inhaling, lower your hands toward the floor and come up leading with relaxed arms and chest.

- Exhaling, lower your arms to your sides. Or pause and bend forward again **(2)**. 3-4x

5.4b — Now that you have loosened up, you can strengthen your back some more.

2. After bending forward, keep your hands on your lower back.

3. Inhaling, come up a little more than half way with your head comfortably back. Pause.

2. Exhaling, bend forward again. Pause. Or, pause and take one breath.

1. Inhaling, come up all the way, leading with your relaxed arms and chest.

3-4x

$$\begin{array}{c}\text{ex} \\ \longrightarrow \\ \longleftarrow \\ \text{in}\end{array}$$

$$\begin{array}{c}\text{in} \\ \longrightarrow \\ \longleftarrow \\ \text{ex}\end{array}$$

➤ *As your back becomes stronger, you might try coming part way up two or even three times in a row before coming up all the way.*

1.  2. 3.

5.4 a

5.4 b

1. Stand with your left foot 2-1/2 to 3-1/2 feet forward. Turn your right foot out slightly.

2. Inhaling, raise your arms from the front, arch your back slightly, and bend your left knee.

3. Exhaling, bend forward placing your hands to either side of your left foot. Take one breath.

2. Inhaling, come up keeping your front knee bent, leading with your arms and chest and arching your back slightly.

• Exhaling, lower your arms from the front and straighten your left leg (1), or pause and bend forward again (3). 3-4x

• Now that you've loosened up, take a breath both in the forward bend (3) and in the arched position with your knee bent (2).

3-4x
Practice the pose equally to the other side.

➤ *If bending your knee in the upright position bothers you, go back to Standing Head to Knee pose (4.3).*

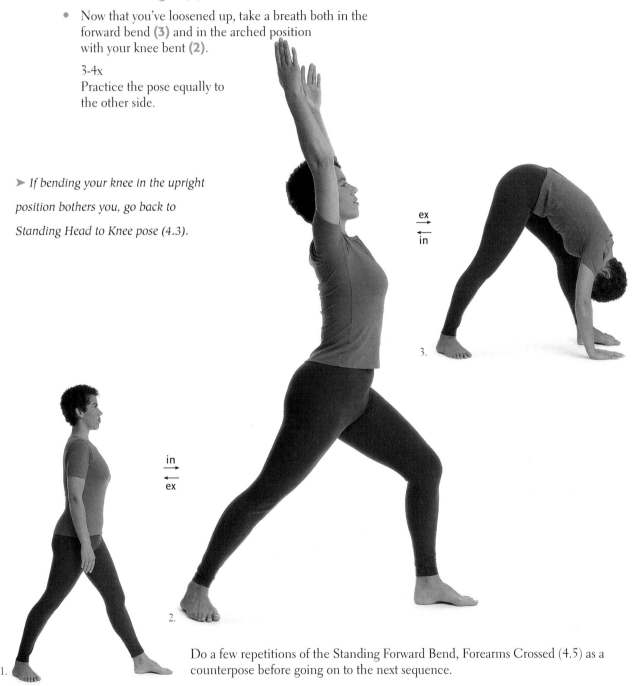

ex
in

in
ex

3.

2.

1.

Do a few repetitions of the Standing Forward Bend, Forearms Crossed (4.5) as a counterpose before going on to the next sequence.

5.6 KNEELING FORWARD BEND UP-AND-DOWN-FACE DOG SEQUENCE

1. Kneel upright, knees slightly apart.

2. Inhaling, raise your arms from the front.

3. Exhaling, bend forward moving your hips back and placing your hands on the floor.

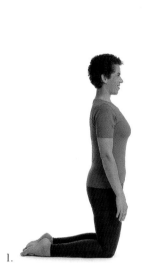

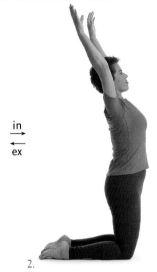

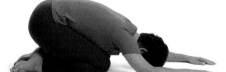

➤ *If you feel strong and comfortable in the sequence, you may go back and forth several times between Up-Face Dog and Down-Face Dog.*

1.   2.   3.

5.7 COBRA WITH ONE BREATH AND 5.8 LOCUST WITH ONE BREATH

1. Lie on your stomach with your legs slightly apart and your arms along-side you, palms up.

2. Inhaling, raise your chest.

1. Exhaling, come down.

   2-3x

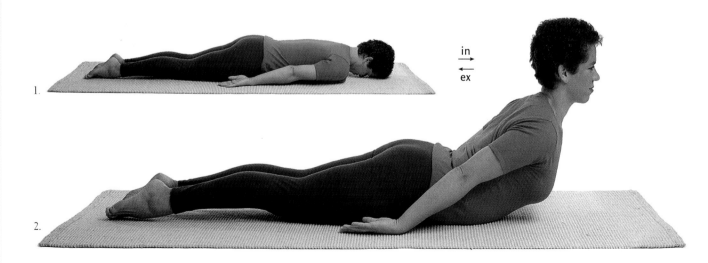

1.

2.

4. Inhaling, move forward into the Up-Face Dog, arching your back and keeping your knees *on* the floor.

5. Exhaling, curl your toes under, lift your hips, and bring your chest toward your knees. Keep your head down and your knees slightly bent in the Down-Face Dog.

Now reverse the sequence:

4. Inhaling, bring your body back to the arched position.

3. Exhaling, return to the kneeling forward bend.

2. Inhaling, come up to an upright kneeling position.

1. Exhaling, lower your arms.

4-6x

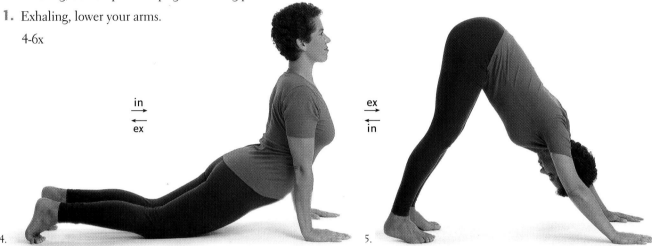

4.

5.

Afterwards lie on your back with your feet flat on the floor and knees up. Slowly raise and lower your arms slowly several times to relax your wrists, arms, shoulders, and lower back.

---

2. Now practice this pose staying up for one breath. Exhaling, lower your head slightly. Inhaling, raise your head slightly and lift your chest a little higher.

1. Exhaling, lower your chest and head to the floor.

2-4x

1 & 3. Follow the same breathing directions in the Locust as you did in the Cobra (5.7), but raise both legs.

2-4x

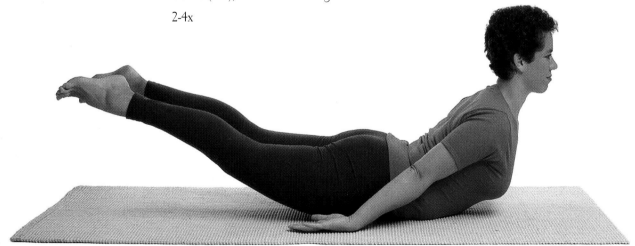

3.

5.9 KNEES TO CHEST POSE (1.5)

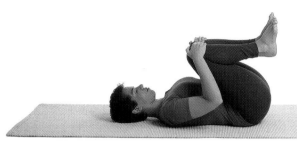

in →
← ex

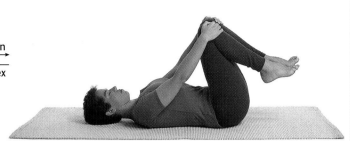

Exhaling, bring your knees toward your chest.

Inhaling, guide your knees away from you.

5.10 LYING DOWN TWIST WITH ONE KNEE BENT (3.9)

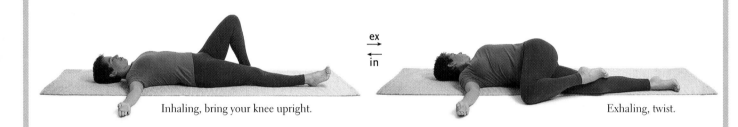

ex →
← in

Inhaling, bring your knee upright.

Exhaling, twist.

5.11 UPWARD LEGS AND ARMS STRETCH (2.9)

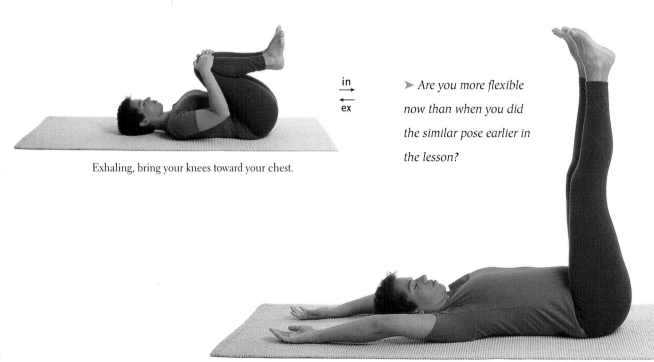

in →
← ex

Exhaling, bring your knees toward your chest.

➤ *Are you more flexible now than when you did the similar pose earlier in the lesson?*

Inhaling, raise your legs and arms.

We finish this lesson with one of our favorite seated breathing exercises, the Caring Breath, aptly named by our students. The arm and head movements combined with the relaxing breath direct your energy inward. You feel soothed and cared for.

1. Sit comfortably on a chair, or cross-legged on a pillow with your back straight. Place your hands on your knees.

- Take a few easy breaths.

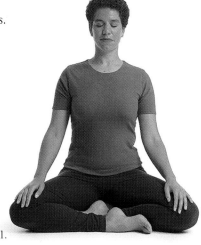

1.

2. Inhaling, raise your right forearm. Pause.

3. Exhaling, turn your head comfortably to the left and bring your right hand to the left side of your chest. Pause.

2. Inhaling, slowly bring your head and forearm to the front.

1. Exhaling, lower your head and right arm. Pause for 1 to 5 seconds. Relax your face and eyes.

- Continue, using your left arm and turning to the right.

- Alternate arms.

- Practice this breath many times.

- Then sit with your face and eyes relaxed and your hands settled comfortably on your knees, abdomen, or chest. Stay relaxed and centered, with your attention deeply inward.

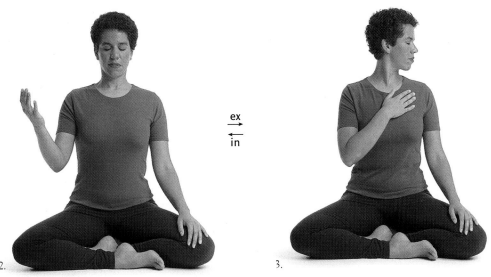

ex →
← in

2.   3.

Rest for 2 minutes, sitting or lying down.

turning yourself

Inversions

This lesson will help you feel how wonderful it is to turn yourself upside down. An inverted posture, such as the Shoulderstand, reverses the effect that gravity has on our bodies over time. Inversions are effective poses for promoting better circulation to the feet, legs, and internal organs. Many of our students comment that practicing inversions gives them a continuous feeling of vitality throughout the day.

Often an inverted pose produces a very calming effect. Students often report that a Shoulderstand quiets their minds and brings their attention inward. Women often tell us that an inversion smoothes out the "jitteriness" and discomfort that may come with ovulation, menstruation, PMS, or menopause. They talk about feeling "in balance" with their hormones and "at ease" after practicing an inverted pose.

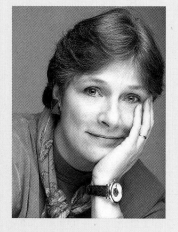

YOGA HELPS A NERVOUS MOTHER-TO-BE THROUGH 12 HOURS OF LABOR

Pam Durban, 48, is the author of a book of short stories, *All Set About with Fever Trees*, and a novel *The Laughing Place*. She teaches at Georgia State: "I started taking yoga at the Pierce Program when I was pregnant. I was 39 and I wanted to do something to stay in shape. It helped me tremendously. After the first trimester I couldn't go a day without doing it. It really strengthened my lower back and gave me a lot of physical confidence. Towards the end of the pregnancy, I was really terrified by the thought of labor. I just wanted to get away from it. I didn't want to go through it. Doing the yoga gave me a feeling of strength. I knew that my body was strong and I was prepared. After practicing the slow breathing for months, I knew I could relax when I needed to. And when the time came, I did. The yoga gave me a sense of control over my body so that I knew what I could do. I had 12 hours of labor, and I never lost control. The yoga, especially the breathing, helped me to focus. It allowed me to relax completely. I really felt I was riding a current."

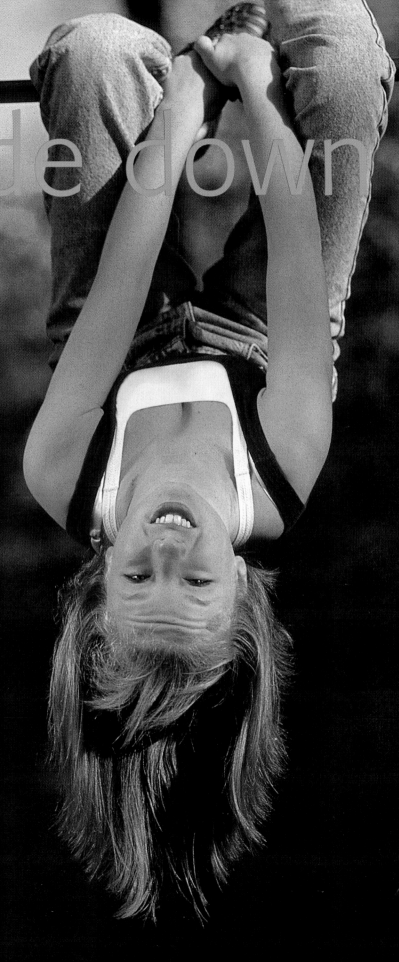

upside down

The Shoulderstand

In the shoulderstand you place your legs above your head and chest and you support your hips with your arms and elbows. This pose requires a strong back, a strong abdomen, and a strong neck. If you have mastered the previous lessons, you should have built sufficient strength and stamina to do the shoulderstand and receive its refreshing benefits. To avoid injuring yourself in the shoulderstand, please prepare thoroughly and afterwards take care of any problems it might have caused by doing all the poses that follow it in this lesson. Proper preparation and proper counter-pose are very important.

It is not necessary, or even always desirable, to have a 'straight' shoulderstand. Please do not force yourself into the vertical position. The important thing is to have your legs above your chest and to breathe deeply and smoothly at a relaxed pace. This will bring you the benefits of the inverted pose.

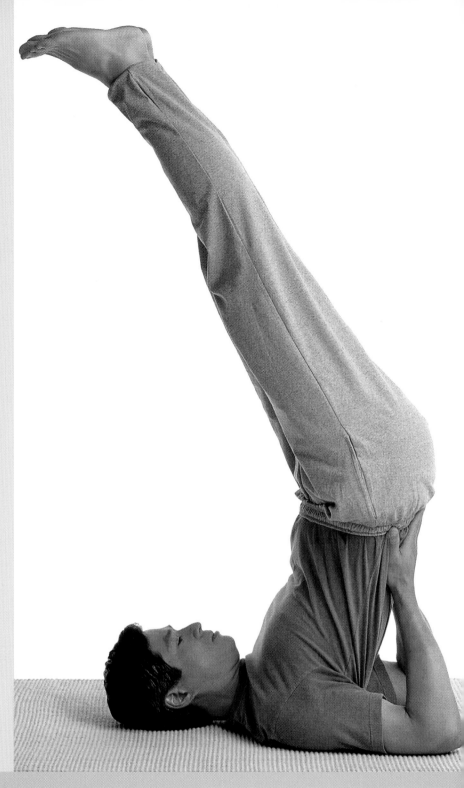

The Shoulderstand Is Not Always for Everyone

The shoulderstand is a wonderful pose, but please approach it with caution. The pose puts a lot of weight on your neck and upper back, which are not designed for such pressure. We urge you not to do it if you have problems in those areas or if you are moderately overweight. You definitely should not do it if you have a hiatal hernia or any neck or back problems that it might aggravate, including: a military neck, a reverse cervical curvature, a whiplash injury, or spinal arthritis.

the 6 lesson

6.1 STANDING FORWARD BEND (1.4, 2.4)

• Practice the pose first pausing in the forward position 4-6x. Then stay in the position while taking a breath. 4-6x

ex →
← in

in →
← ex

Inhaling, raise your arms.   Exhaling, bend forward.   Inhaling, arch your back.

6.2 TRIANGLE (2.3), THEN TRIANGLE TWIST TO CENTER (4.4)

• Start by loosening up with the Triangle (2.3).
  3-4x per side, alternating sides.

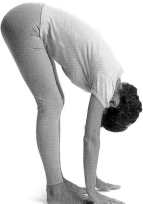

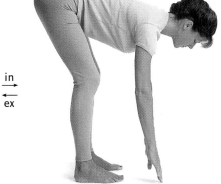

ex →
← in

Inhaling, raise your arms from the side.   Exhaling, turn and bring your right hand to your left foot.

• Then go on to the more demanding Triangle Twist to Center (4.4).

3-4x per side, alternating sides.

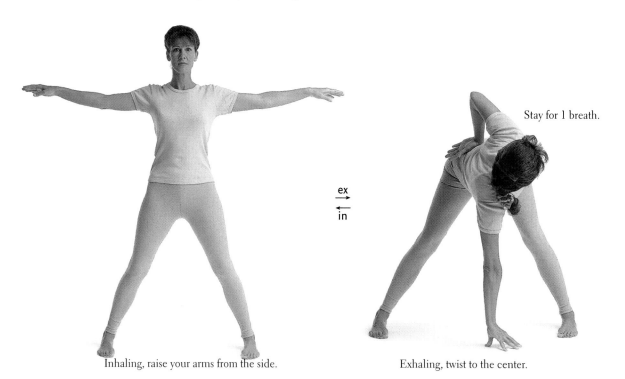

Stay for 1 breath.

ex
→
←
in

Inhaling, raise your arms from the side.   Exhaling, twist to the center.

➤ *After you have loosened up, if staying one breath in the twisted position feels fine, try staying for two breaths.*

6.3 STANDING FORWARD BEND SWEEPING ARMS

AND COMING UP PART WAY (5.4a&b)

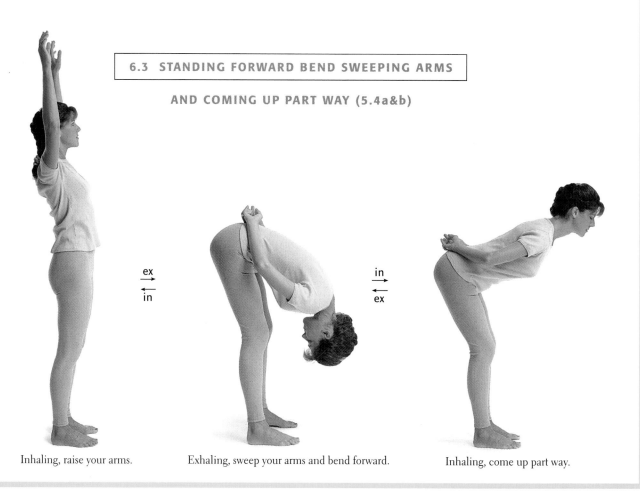

ex
→
←
in

in
→
←
ex

Inhaling, raise your arms.   Exhaling, sweep your arms and bend forward.   Inhaling, come up part way.

KNEES OFF THE FLOOR

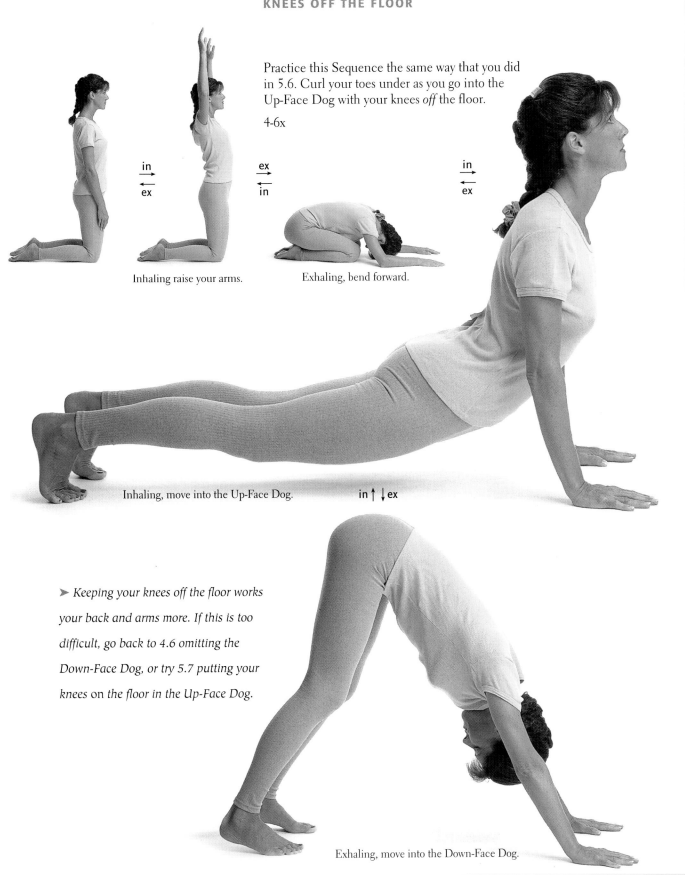

Practice this Sequence the same way that you did in 5.6. Curl your toes under as you go into the Up-Face Dog with your knees *off* the floor.

4-6x

in → ← ex

Inhaling raise your arms.

ex → ← in

Exhaling, bend forward.

in → ← ex

Inhaling, move into the Up-Face Dog.

in ↑ ↓ ex

➤ *Keeping your knees off the floor works your back and arms more. If this is too difficult, go back to 4.6 omitting the Down-Face Dog, or try 5.7 putting your knees on the floor in the Up-Face Dog.*

Exhaling, move into the Down-Face Dog.

Practice as in 1.3, but take one breath *in the floor position* as well as in the arch. The extra breath will help relax your back in preparation for the Shoulderstand.

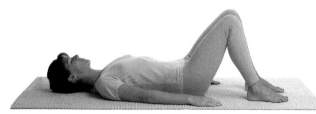 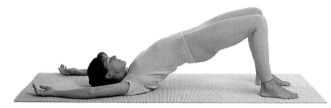 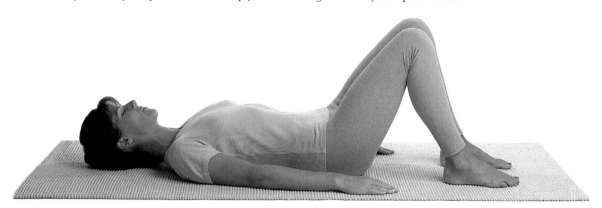

Exhaling, lower your arms and hip.   Inhaling, raise your arms and hips.

6.6 SHOULDERSTAND

1. Lie on your back, with your knees up and your feet flat on the floor. Bring your arms close to you with your palms down. Keep your head aligned with your spine. Inhale.

2. Exhaling, raise your legs and hips off the floor and slowly swing your legs behind you over your head.

> ➤ *If you have no neck problems, a strong back, and strong abdominals, you may start with your legs together, straight out on the floor. Otherwise start with your knees up, feet flat on the floor.*

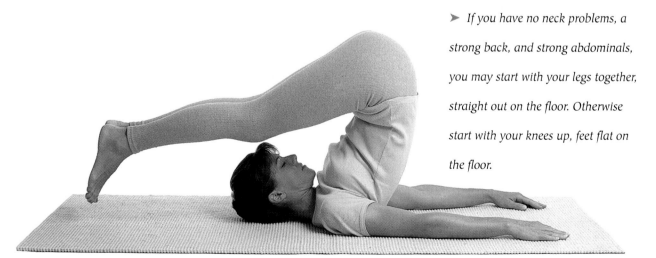

3. Inhaling, support your lower back with your hands and raise your legs, straightening your body. Avoid forcing up farther than is comfortable. A straight vertical position can hurt your neck. How far you staighten up will depend on your particular body.

- Stay 4-6 breaths.

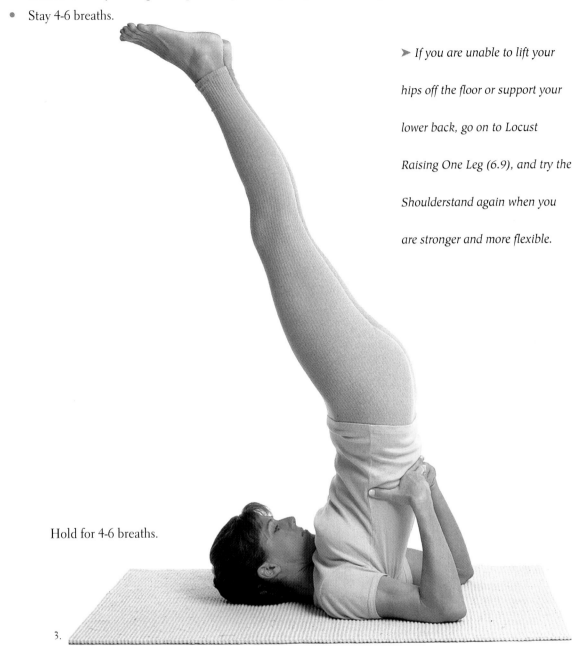

➤ *If you are unable to lift your hips off the floor or support your lower back, go on to Locust Raising One Leg (6.9), and try the Shoulderstand again when you are stronger and more flexible.*

Hold for 4-6 breaths.

3.

4. To come down, exhaling, lower your legs behind you and bring your arms onto the floor, palms down.

5. Inhaling, lower your hips to the floor.

6. Exhaling, bring your knees toward your chest and rest.

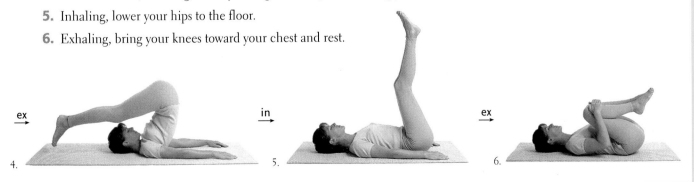

ex →   in →   ex →

4.   5.   6.

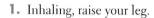

6.7 SHOULDERSTAND WITH KNEE LOWERING

If the Shoulderstand felt comfortable, practice knee lowerings.

1. Go up into the Shoulderstand.

• Take one or two breaths as you stay in the pose.

2. Exhaling, bend one knee toward your ear.

1. Inhaling, raise your leg.

• Alternate lowering each leg several times, then come down to the floor as in 6.6 to rest.

3-4x per leg.

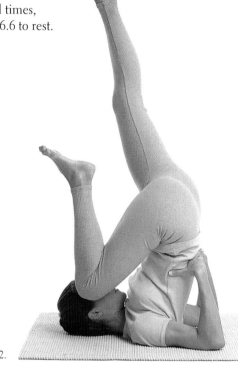

1.   2.

Adapting Shoulderstand

If your Shoulderstand is wobbly or difficult, try practicing a partial Shoulderstand with your feet against the wall for support.

You may want to ask a teacher to check your alignment in the Shoulderstand.

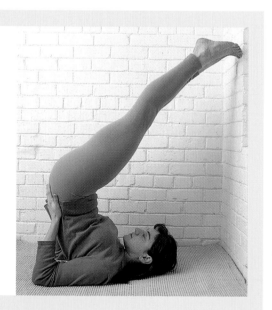

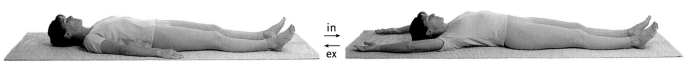

Exhaling, lower your arms.　　　　　　　　　　　　Inhaling, raise your arms.

➤ *You may practice this with legs straight, as shown, or knees bent. Depending on how your body feels today you might also want to do a few repetitions of the Cat (1.7), or Bridge (1.3) or Knees to Chest Pose (1.5) before going on to the Cobra/Locust variations.*

6.9 LOCUST RAISING ONE LEG AND BOTH LEGS

1. Lie on your stomach, legs slightly apart, arms at your sides, palms up.

2. Inhaling, raise your chest and head into the Cobra (4.9).

1-2x

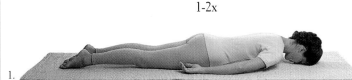

1.

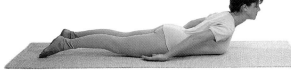

2.

1 & 3. Now practice the Locust Raising One Leg,

1-2x raising the left leg, then 1-2x raising the right leg.

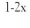

3.

1 & 4. Next practice the Locust raising both legs (4.10).

1-2x

• Now that you have loosened up in all three versions, practice them taking one breath in the arch. This is demanding, but it is a wonderful back strengthener!

1-2x

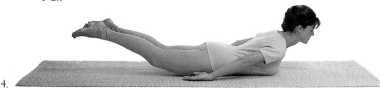

4.

6.10 KNEES TO CHEST POSE (1.5)

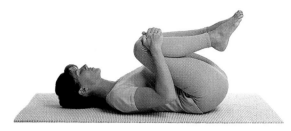

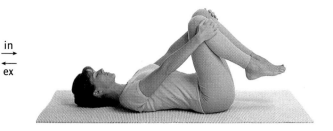

Exhaling, bring your knees toward your chest.

Inhaling, guide your knees away from you.

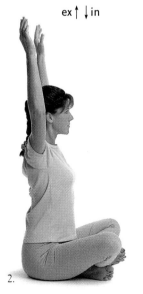

6.11 SEATED CROSS-LEGGED FORWARD BEND

1. Sit with your legs crossed and your arms and shoulders relaxed.

2. Inhaling, raise your arms from the front.

3. Exhaling, bend forward. Rest your arms with your elbows bent on the floor.

4. Take one breath. Inhaling, keep your hands on the floor and arch until your arms are straight.

3. Exhaling, bend down again.

2. Inhaling, come up leading with your arms and chest.

3. Go forward again and take two breaths. If that feels good, continue, taking two or even three breaths in the forward bend.

4-5x

ex ↑ ↓ in

> *If your knees are higher than your hips, you may need to sit on a small pillow. If you have knee problems or if this pose is uncomfortable, skip it and go on to the next pose. Try it again in a few months when you've loosened up more.*

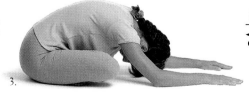

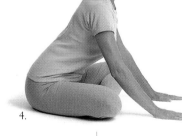

Repeat
Stay for 1, 2, and 3 breaths.

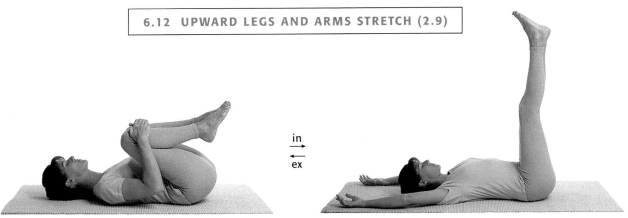

in
ex

Exhaling, bring your knees toward your chest.

Inhaling, raise your legs and arms.

6.13 PROGRESSIVE BREATHING

- Sit on a chair or a pillow with your legs comfortably relaxed. Or lie down in one of the rest positions.
- Inhale for 3 seconds. Pause. Exhale for 3 seconds. Pause.
- Continue to follow the pattern outlined below, gradually extending your breath. Practice each breath count one or two times.

IN Pause	EX Pause
3 sec.	3 sec.
4	4
5	5
6	6
6	7
6	8
6	9
6	10
then	reverse

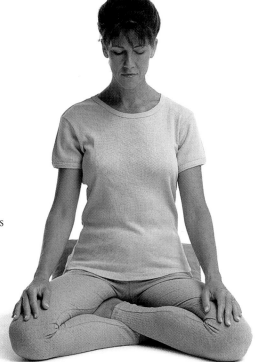

- When you reverse the sequence, gradually shorten the exhalations, and then gradually shorten your inhalations and exhalations until you are once again inhaling 3 seconds and exhaling 3 seconds. Continue with that easy 3/3 pattern until you just want to rest.

  The numbers here are only an approximate guide. Perhaps you will go to a 5-7, or an 8-16 maximum. Breathe without strain.

  Rest for 2 minutes, or for as long as you like.

You can learn each lesson at your own pace. Practice as often and for as many weeks as you like. You can go back to previous lessons if they are particularly enjoyable to you. But be sure that you can do the poses in this lesson with confidence before moving on.

a longer, challenging

CONCEPTS & PRINCIPLES

Having mastered the relaxing poses of the first lessons, you are now ready for the more demanding poses in this workout. To raise your energy level, first warm up and loosen your muscles with the Standing Forward Bend. Use this pose to begin to slow your breath and focus your mind. Afterwards, you will be ready to do the more vigorous poses that are the core of this lesson. You should enjoy the feelings of alertness and strength that come with the workout. The last few poses are simple and quiet in order to cool you down, steady your breathing, and focus your mind.

As with all yoga poses, try to maintain slow, even breathing in the workout. Maintaining a steady and smooth breath makes the poses more effective and challenging and ensures that you are practicing safely. Your breath indicates whether you are ready to do the pose or whether you are pushing yourself too much. If your breath becomes ragged, or if you feel that you are straining, pause and rest for at least a few breaths. If you are too tired or tense to relax, we urge you to go back to a less demanding lesson. Otherwise, this lesson might increase your tension.

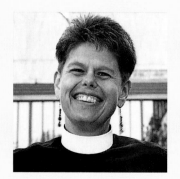

YOGA ENRICHES LIFE FOR AN ATHLETIC PRIEST

Bobbie Patterson, Ph.D., 43, is an Episcopal priest and Assistant Professor of Religion at Emory University: "I do very rigorous and regular disciplined athletic activities. These include squash, biking, swimming, and weight lifting. Yoga is an antidote for the damage I might do to myself with these other exercises. It keeps me limber so that I am less likely to hurt myself. Yoga has been very important in my spiritual life, as well. It has helped me experience what all spiritual teachings tell us: that the soul and the body are one. The breath of life, as I experience it in yoga, makes me feel whole–physically, mentally, and spiritually. I've come to understand how to use breathing to look inside of me, to find a center in myself, and to connect with God or the universal power."

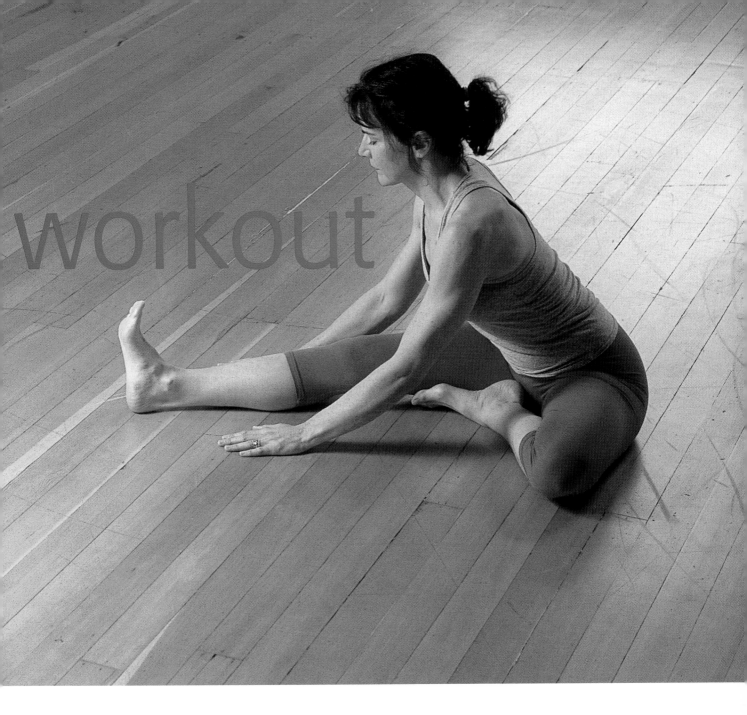

workout

In this lesson you will find new variations of poses you have done in previous lessons. We have changed the poses slightly so that they help strengthen your back. In some of the poses, we change the pattern of breathing, asking you to stay in the pose for several breaths, thereby increasing the challenge. As always, if any of the poses cause you pain, we urge you to stop and do the easier variations or adaptations.

the lesson 7

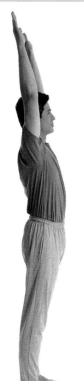

Practice between 4-8 repetitions. Can you now feel the effects that the repetitive movements have on your body?

7.1 STANDING FORWARD BEND (1.4, 2.4)

ex
→
←
in

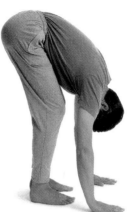

in
→
←
ex

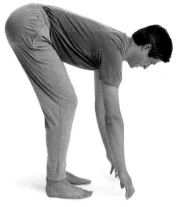

Inhaling, raise your arms.

Exhaling, bend forward.

Inhaling, arch your back slightly.

7.2 STANDING BACK ARCH (5.5)

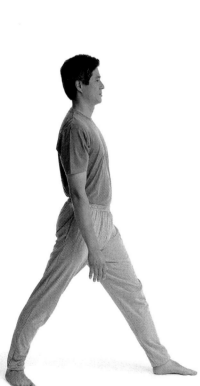

in
→
←
ex

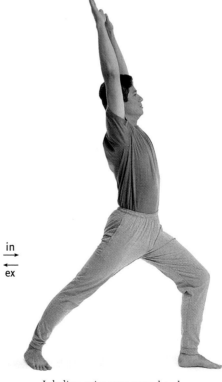

ex
→
←
in

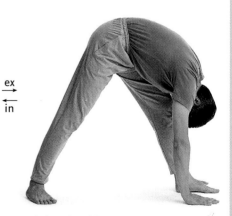

Stand with your feet apart.

Inhaling, raise your arms, bend your forward knee, and arch your back.

Exhaling, bend forward into the Head-to-Knee pose. Practice both sides equally.

AND COMING UP PART-WAY LEADING WITH ONE ARM

1 & 2. Practice the Standing Forward Bend (1.4) as a counterpose to the Standing Back Arch. 3-4 x

2. Then bring your feet a little further apart. Exhaling, bend forward again.

3. Inhaling, bend your knees a bit more and come one-half to two-thirds of the way up, leading with your right arm. Keep it relaxed. Place your left hand near your left knee. Pause a few seconds allowing your back to work more.

2. Exhaling, bend forward again.

3. Inhaling, come up part way leading with your other arm. Pause a few seconds.

2. Exhaling, bend down straightening your legs somewhat. Take one breath in the forward bend. Relax your back, shoulders, and neck.

1. Inhaling, come all the way up leading with your arms and chest.

• Pause. Exhaling, continue with another forward bend, or lower your arms.

Repeat the sequence 3-4x.

1.

ex
→
←
in

2.

in
→
←
ex

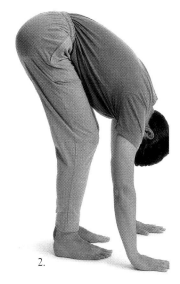

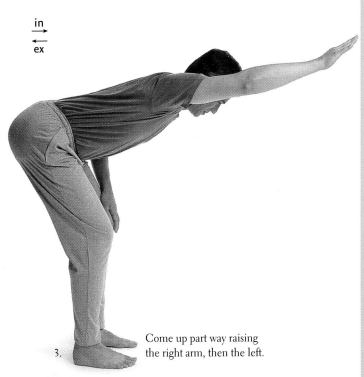

➤ *If this pose bothers your back, try an easier version of the Standing Forward Bend such as 2.4. On the other hand, if you want to make the pose more challenging, after loosening up, try coming up part way two or three times in a row with each arm. Remember to take a breath in the forward bend, relaxing your lower back before coming up all the way.*

3.   Come up part way raising the right arm, then the left.

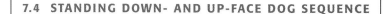

1. Stand with your feet 6 to 12 inches apart.

2. Inhaling, raise your arms from the front.

3. Exhaling, bend forward placing your hands on the floor, and step back 3 to 3-1/2 feet, one leg at a time, bringing your chest toward your knees. Keep your head relaxed down and your knees slightly bent in the Down-Face Dog.

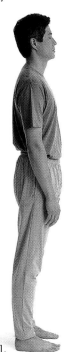

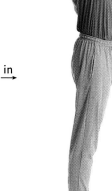

in →

ex →

in →

1.

2.

3.

5. Exhaling, press your toes, lift your hips, and lower your head, returning to the Down-Face Dog. Inhale and stay in place.

6-7. Exhaling, step forward one leg at a time bringing your feet toward your hands, feet parallel, 6 to 12 inches apart. Take a breath if you need to.

Inhale and stay.

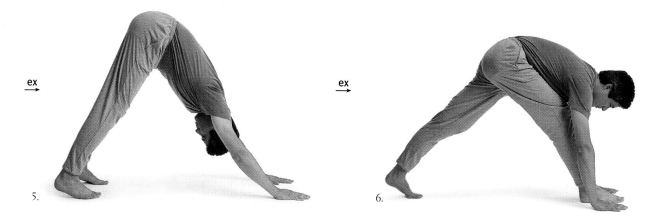

ex →

ex →

5.

6.

Exhaling, step forward first with one foot, then with the other foot.

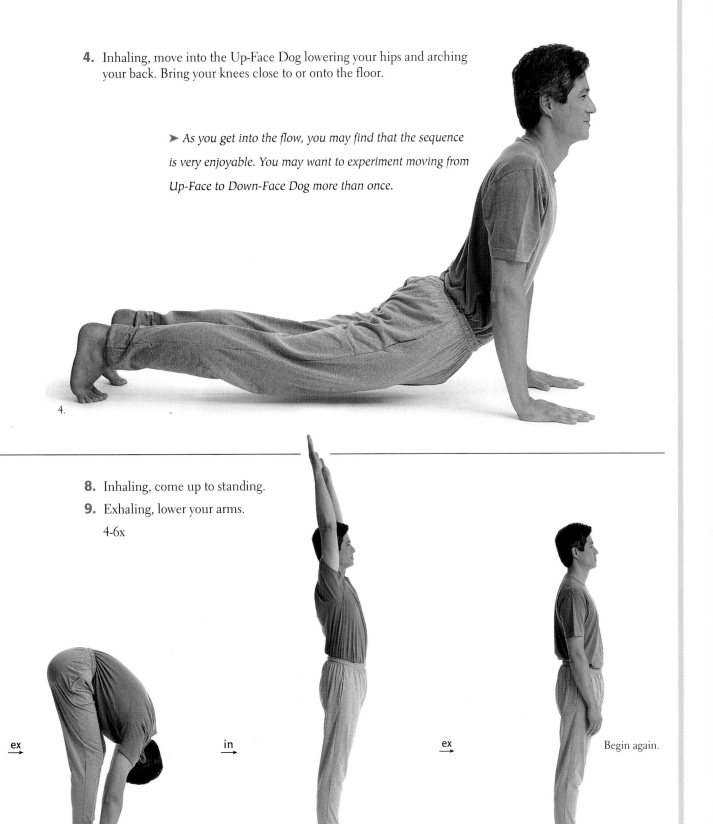

4. Inhaling, move into the Up-Face Dog lowering your hips and arching your back. Bring your knees close to or onto the floor.

> ➤ *As you get into the flow, you may find that the sequence is very enjoyable. You may want to experiment moving from Up-Face to Down-Face Dog more than once.*

4.

8. Inhaling, come up to standing.

9. Exhaling, lower your arms.

4-6x

ex →

7.

in →

8.

ex →

9.

Begin again.

Sit or walk in place. When your breath is back to a normal easy rhythm, go on to the next pose.

7.5 SIDE STRETCH WITH FOOT TURNED

1. Stand with your feet 2-1/2 to 3-1/2 feet apart. Turn your left foot so that your left heel points to your right instep.

2. Inhaling, raise your arms from the side to shoulder level.

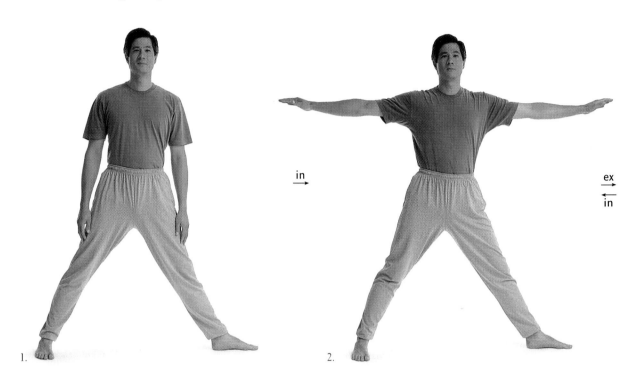

in →

ex →
← in

1.

2.

7.6 STANDING FORWARD BEND, FOREARMS CROSSED (4.5)

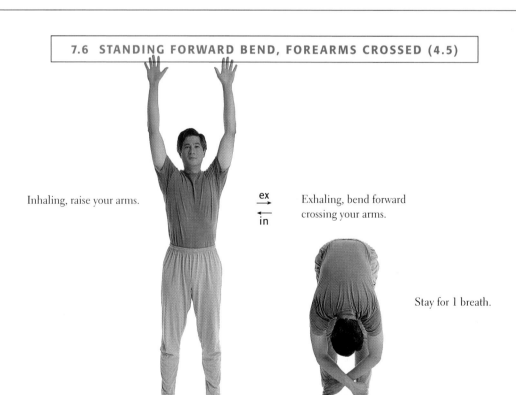

Inhaling, raise your arms.

ex →
← in

Exhaling, bend forward crossing your arms.

Stay for 1 breath.

3. Exhaling, guide your left hand down your left leg, and hold firmly near your left ankle. Keep your head and right arm relaxed.

4. Inhaling, reach to the side with your right arm. Keep your arm slightly bent and relaxed.

3. Exhaling, bring your arm up and out from your right shoulder again.

2. Inhaling, come up. Pause, bringing your feet parallel.

• Exhaling, change your foot position and stretch to the right side.

   Repeat 3-5x per side, alternating sides.

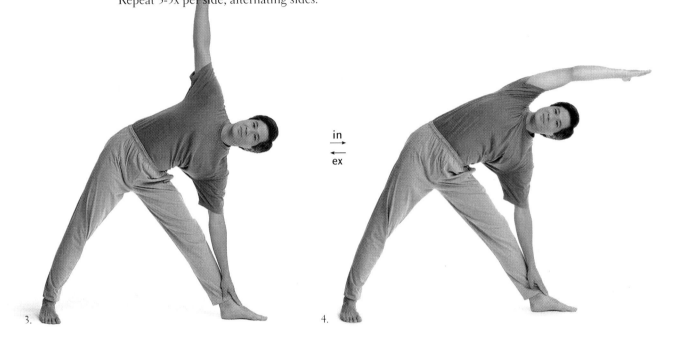

7.7 BRIDGE (1.3)

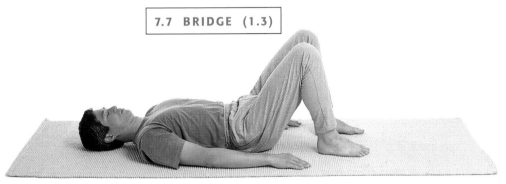

Exhaling, lower your arms and hips.

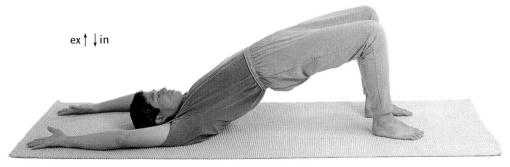

Inhaling, raise your arms and hips.

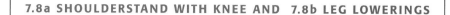

7.8a First work the Shoulderstand with Knee Lowerings:

1. Move into Shoulderstand (6.6) and stay for several breaths.

2. Then add the Shoulderstand with Knee Lowering (6.7).

2x each knee, alternating.

ex →
← in

7.8b Then work in the Shoulderstand with Leg Lowerings:

3. Exhaling, lower one leg toward the floor. Keep your leg straight. Pause.

1. Inhaling, raise your leg.

3-4x each leg, alternating.

ex
in

➤ *If this pose is too difficult for you or causes you discomfort, skip it and go on to the Cobra/Locust (7.10).*

Adapting the Shoulderstand with Knee and Leg Lowerings

If you are strong and limber, try this variation for more challenge:

1. Exhaling, bend your right knee toward your right ear. Pause.

2 & 3. Inhaling, first straighten your right leg and bring your right foot toward or to the floor. Continue to inhale, raising your straight leg up to join your left leg.

3-4x per leg, alternating.

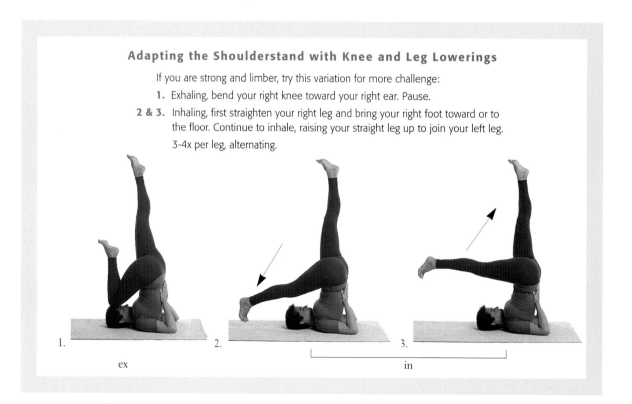

ex

in

7.9 ARM RAISE (1.1)

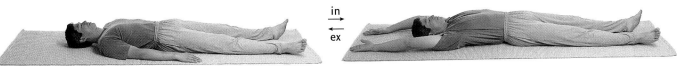

Exhaling, lower your arms.

Inhaling, raise your arms.

➤ *Feel free to practice some Cat, Bridge, or Knees to Chest Pose if you need to before proceeding to the Cobra/Locust variations.*

7.10 COBRA/LOCUST WITH ARM MOVEMENTS

Begin with the simple Cobra pose.

1. Lie on your front, legs slightly apart, arms along-side you, palms up.

2. Inhaling, raise your chest and tip your head slightly back.

1. Exhaling, lower back down to the floor.

2x

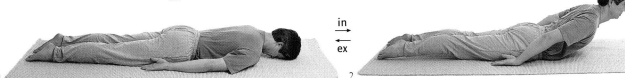

Add arm and leg movements.

3. Inhaling, raise your chest and left leg as you sweep your right arm off the floor to the side and forward. Tip your head back slightly.

1. Exhaling, lower yourself to the floor, sweeping your arm alongside you again.

• Practice the same pattern, now raising your right leg and left arm.

2x each side, alternating.

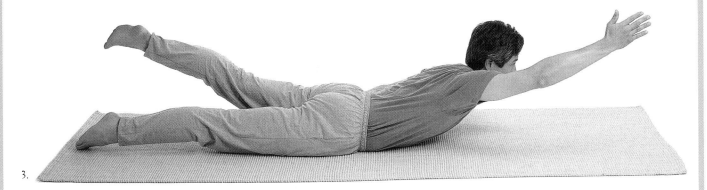

Now you are ready to raise both arms and both legs.

4. Inhaling, raise your chest and both legs, and sweep both arms off the floor to the front of your head.

1. Exhaling, lower yourself to the floor, sweeping your arms back along-side you again.

2x

• Repeat all three pose variations, while staying for one breath in each of the arching positions.

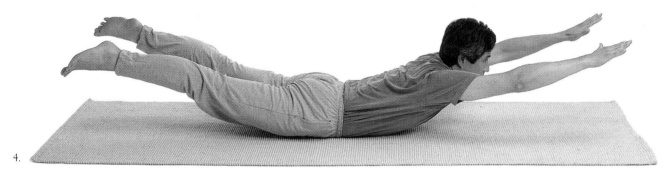

4.

➤ *If you feel strong in these poses, try staying for two breaths in the arch position. But if staying up makes you feel tense or bothers your back, skip the extra breaths. As in all Cobra/Locust poses, move your head only slightly. Avoid compressing in the back of your neck. Let your back do the work. Rest with your head to the side whenever you need to.*

Before moving on to the following counterpose, relax on your stomach with your head turned to the left for a couple of easy breaths. Then turn your head to the right for a few breaths.

7.11 KNEES TO CHEST POSE (1.5)

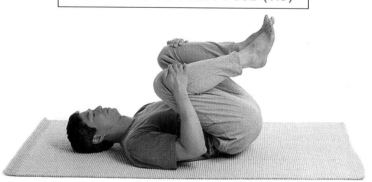

Exhaling, bring your knees toward your chest.

ex ↑ ↓ in

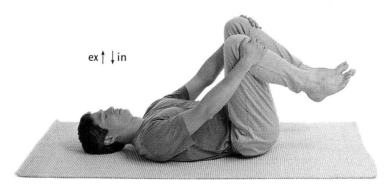

Inhaling, guide your knees away from you.

7.12 SEATED HEAD TO KNEE POSE

1. Sit on the floor. Bring your left leg straight out in front of you. Place the sole of your right foot against your left upper thigh.

2. Inhaling, raise your arms from the front.

3. Exhaling, bend forward toward your left leg. Keep your arms bent, shoulders and head relaxed, and place your hands on your leg.

4. Inhaling, keep your hands on your leg and arch up part way. Lengthen your spine and straighten your arms.

3. Exhaling, relax down into the stretch again.

2. Inhaling, come up all the way, leading with your arms and chest.

• Repeat several times. Then try staying forward (3) for 2 to 3 breaths.

• Practice equally to the other leg.

3-5x per leg.

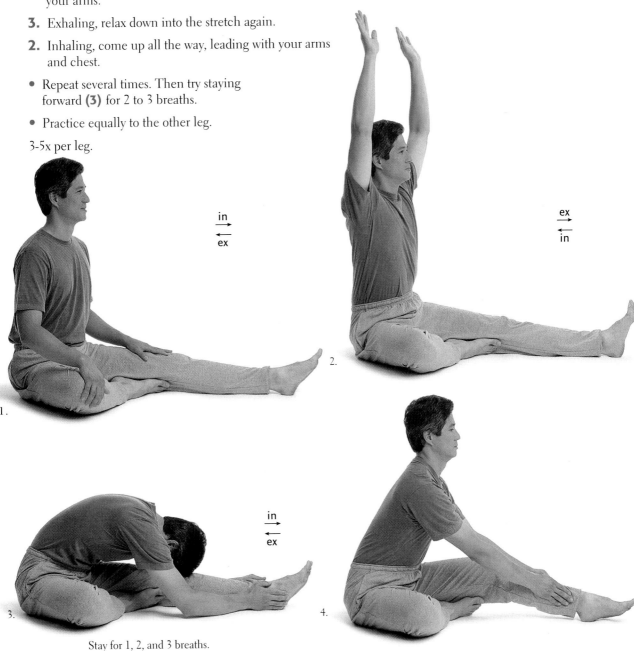

in
ex

ex
in

in
ex

Stay for 1, 2, and 3 breaths.

➤ *If your leg or back is tight, sit on a pillow or two. You can also put a small pillow under the knee of your straight leg. If these changes don't make this pose more comfortable, go on to the next pose.*

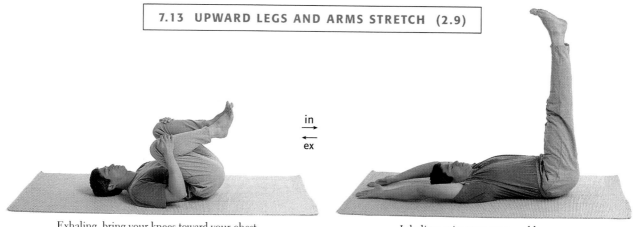

Exhaling, bring your knees toward your chest.

Inhaling, raise your arms and legs.

7.14 SEATED PALMING

- Sit comfortably on a chair or pillow, with your back straight and shoulders relaxed. Take a few easy breaths.

2. Exhaling, lower your head as you bring your hands to your eyes. Lightly palm your eyes. Take a breath, comfortably extending your exhalation.

1. Inhaling, slowly lower your hands, palming them together as you bring your head slightly back.

2. Exhaling, lower your head, palm your eyes again and take a breath.

- Bring your attention more and more deeply inward with each breath. Continue to relax your face and eyes as you exhale. Feel a quiet energy, a calm inner strength. Continue the Seated Palming until you want to sit or lie down for a few minutes with your eyes closed.

10-20 Breaths

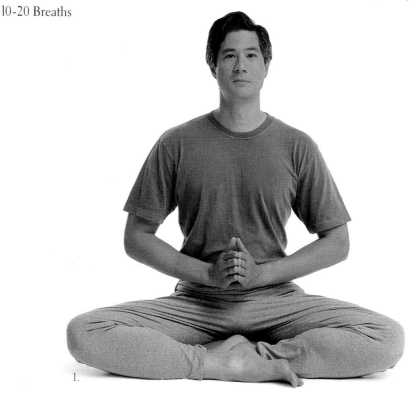

1.

ex
in

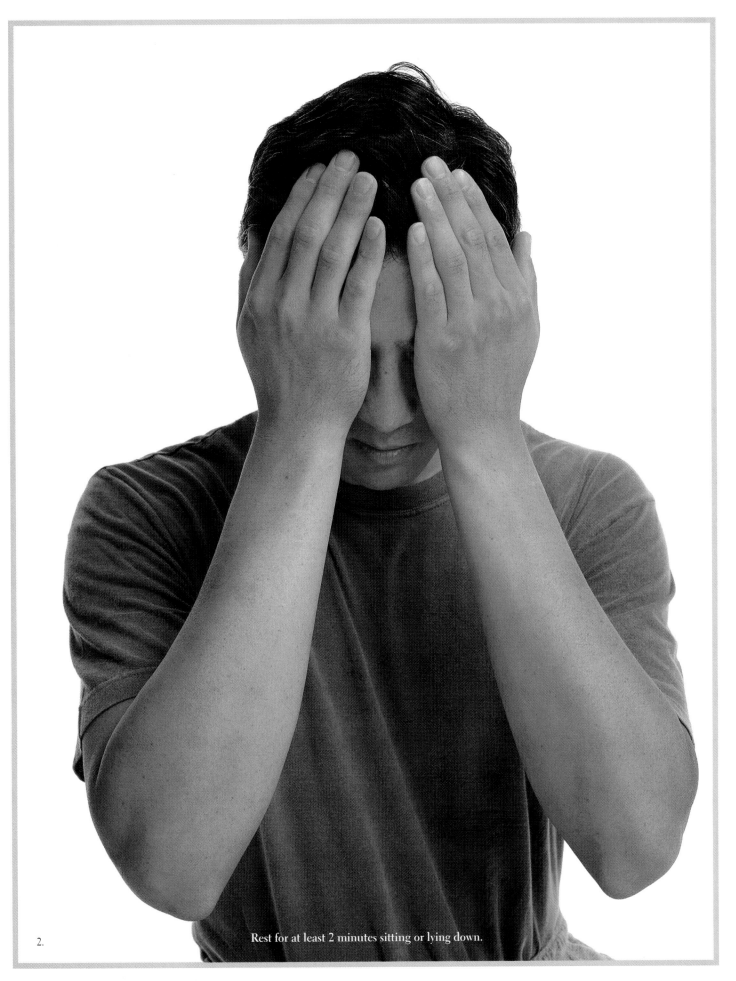

2.

Rest for at least 2 minutes sitting or lying down.

moving in

CONCEPTS & PRINCIPLES

Dynamic Sequences

A dynamic sequence (*vinyasa* in Sanskrit) links poses together, forming a rhythmic fluid dance. By building on basic yoga poses you can make flowing transitions from one pose to the next. You can design an endless number of dynamic sequences. Some will be vigorous workouts, some will emphasize stretching, and others will focus on quiet relaxation. A *vinyasa* combines poses for a complete well-rounded workout of all the major muscle groups of the body. A great way to start the day!

Sometimes you won't have time to do the slow, careful programs we have presented so far. These may be times to do a short dynamic sequence. A continuous flow of poses can quickly give you overall stretch, strength, and focus. A dynamic sequence will help you to concentrate, especially if you have to practice with distractions nearby. Parents with infants and small children in the house often find *vinyasas* helpful. If you're feeling stressed, anxious, or depressed, a sequence may quickly bring you calmness and inner strength. A vigorous *vinyasa* can also be an enjoyable way to get a good workout with a lot of strong stretching when you don't have much time. You can do each sequence several times or only once.

As you practice a sequence, you can become immersed into the rhythm of your movement and breathing. Each inhalation and exhalation is like a wave expanding and contracting your body. You tune into your own inner flow. As you practice these sequences, establish a steady, even pace of movement and breathing. As you become attuned to this rhythm, you may begin to notice a sense of quiet or stillness that links all the movements together. Let yourself become absorbed into that calm state.

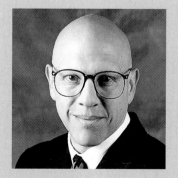

A TOP REPORTER'S COPING WEAPON

Art Harris, an award-winning TV correspondent, recalls how he drew on yoga as part of his 'psychic survival kit': "I was sent to do a story for the *Washington Post* about a fugitive tax evader who was gunned down while holed up in this little mountain cabin after killing a sheriff in rural Arkansas. I'd had only three hours sleep the night before, driving two or three hours up into the mountains. Then I had only an hour on the ground to gather information and interview people. I had to rush back to a sleazy little motel and write. The only way I was able to make my deadline and write the story was to do energizing yoga breathing. It woke me up, cleared my mind, and helped me to concentrate. For me, yoga is an extra coping weapon. I use it to help me survive the unexpected and cope while exploring the thicket of life."

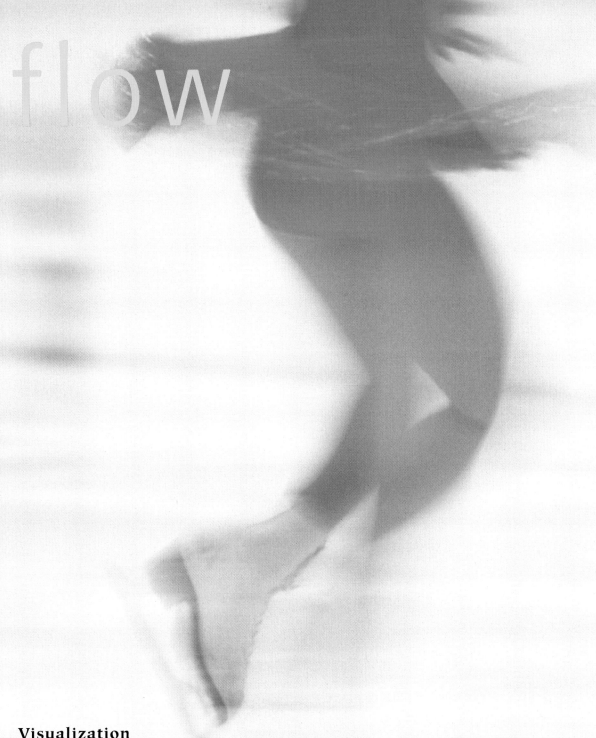

f l o w

Visualization

Vizualization is a powerful yoga method that western medical science has only recently begun to appreciate. If you imagine bringing healing energy into your body, you will very likely feel better. Students of ours have used visualizations in combination with yoga poses, breathing, and orthodox and unorthodox treatments to influence and better manage the course of "intractable" diseases, such as cancer. Their doctors have sometimes been surprised at how well they have done.

I, Margaret, use a positive image when I want to heal myself. Sometimes, I lie next to a window and feel the sun's warmth. Often I touch the area that I want to take care of, or I imagine myself touching

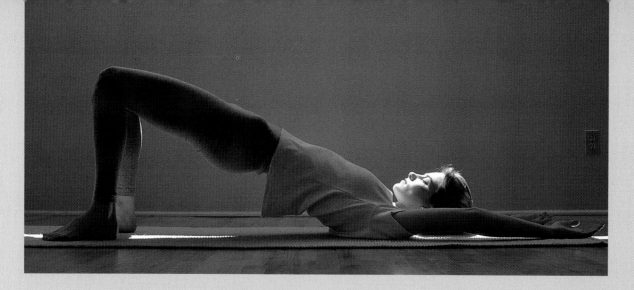

it. With slow, easy breathing I visualize bathing the area in a warm healing, white, yellow, or golden light. It helps me. You might try using visualization to speed up the healing of a sore throat or to alleviate a headache.

Through purposeful visualization you can often change your mind, emotions, and behavior in a powerful way. For instance before I, Martin, teach a class, I sit and take some easy breaths. Then I visualize compassion—first for myself and then for the person or group that I plan to teach. Inhaling, I bring my hands to my heart and think of taking care of myself. Exhaling, I bring my hands to my knees and imagine myself letting go of the tensions that sometimes keep me from being with others in a friendly, open way. After I have done this for a while and feel that I have taken care of myself, I keep my hands on my heart, and I think of the person or people that I plan to teach in a caring way. Afterwards I feel that I am more attentive to my students. I feel freer, more intuitive, and better able to give them what they need.

We teach a yoga visualization which helps many people:

• Imagine that somewhere in your abdomen you have a fire or a small furnace.

• Then picture everything mental and physical that you don't need—sickness, aches, pains, anxiety, depression—as a kind of mass located below the fire.

• Visualize that each inhalation blows a little of this unneeded stuff into the fire and burns it up.

• Each exhalation blows a little of it off as ash.

Imagine that with each breath you purify and refine your mind and body. After this visualization you may find yourself revitalized.

There are visualizations for every conceivable situation or problem. To be effective they need to be adapted to your personality and situation. Be imaginative. Find the one or ones that feel right for you.

To get you started, we suggest a visualization at the end of this lesson which many people have found soothing and refreshing. Use it to care for yourself.

the 8 lesson

8.1 STANDING FORWARD BEND (1.4)

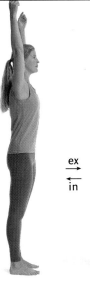
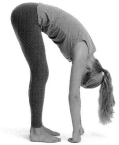

Inhaling, raise your arms.   Exhaling, bend forward.

Adapting the Standing Combination

You can make the sequence on the following pages
more demanding by substituting the following adaptations:

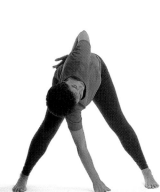

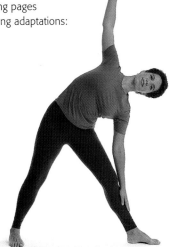

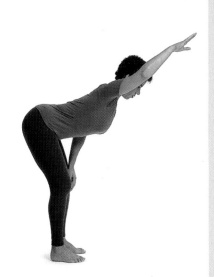

Triangle Twist to Center (4.4),   **Side Stretch with Foot Turned (7.5),**   or **the Standing Forward Bend Coming Up Part Way Leading with One Arm (7.3).**

Or you can make the sequence longer and more varied by doing the easier variation immediately followed by the more difficult one.

When you are comfortable with the basic sequence, have fun making up your own individualized sequence with these variations!

The first dynamic sequence in this lesson is made up of poses you have already learned in Lessons 1 - 7. Notice that you will counterpose the Twist and Side Stretch with a Forward Bend.

1. Stand with your feet well apart and your arms and shoulders relaxed by your sides.

2. Inhaling, raise your arms from the front.

3. Exhaling, bend forward. Take one breath (as in 2.4, except place your feet well apart to anticipate the next poses).

4. Inhaling, come up raising your arms from the side to shoulder level.

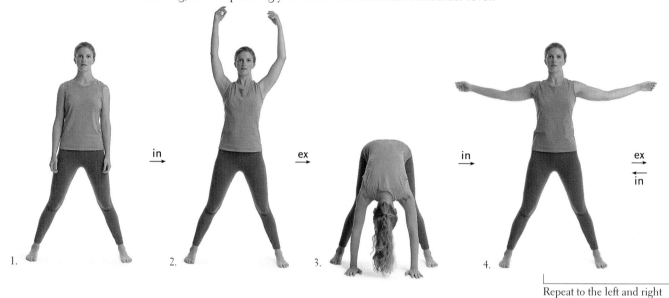

Repeat to the left and right

9. Exhaling, stretch to the left side, placing your left hand on your leg.

10. Inhaling, reach to the left with your right arm.

9. Exhaling, raise your arm up toward the ceiling.

11. Inhaling, come up bringing your arms to shoulder level.

● Repeat to the right side.

12. Exhaling, bend forward to counterpose the side stretch. Take one breath.

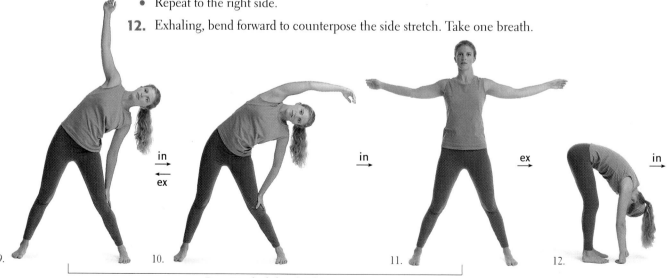

Repeat to the left and right

5 & 4. Exhaling, move into the Triangle Twist to Side (3.3). Take one breath. Inhaling, come up. Exhaling, twist to the other side. Take one breath.

6. Inhaling, come up raising your arms from the side to shoulder level.

7. Exhaling, bend forward into the Standing Forward Bend Forearms Crossed (4.5) to counterpose. Take one breath in the down position.

8. Inhaling, come up, raising your arms from the side to shoulder level.

➤ *Watch your breathing in this and the following sequences. If your breath becomes ragged or strained, stop and take an extra breath. Then continue.*

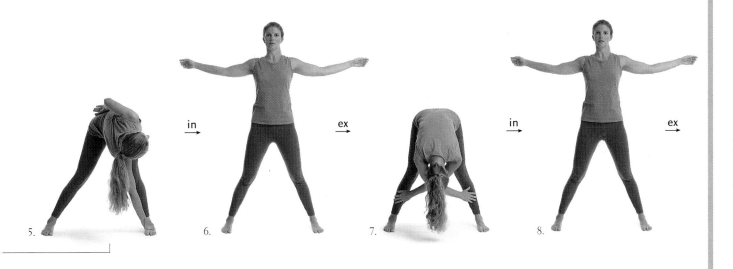

5.   in →   6.   ex →   7.   in →   8.   ex →

13. Inhaling, come up raising your arms overhead.

14. Exhaling, bend forward sweeping your arms to the side and onto your lower back.

15. Inhaling, come up part way.

16. Exhaling, bend forward again.

17. Inhaling, lower your arms and then come all the way up leading with your arms and chest.

18. Exhaling, lower your arms to your sides.

Repeat the entire sequence 1-4x.

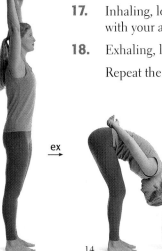
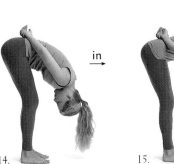
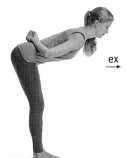
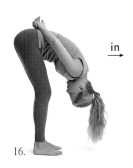
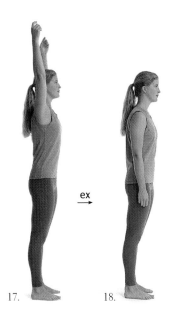

13.   ex →   14.   in →   15.   ex →   16.   in →   17.   18.   ex →

In this next dynamic sequence we introduce a new pose called the Stick. This sequence is a continuous combination, where the second half is simply the reverse of the first half.

1. Kneel upright with your arms by your sides.

2. Inhaling, raise your arms.

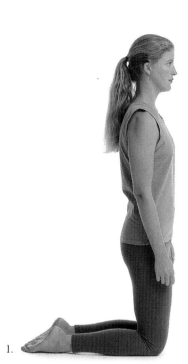

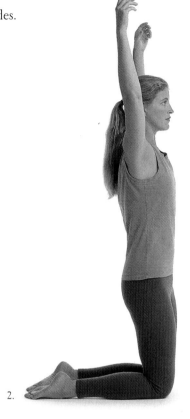

in →
← ex

ex →
← in

1.

2.

5. Exhaling, curl your toes under, raise your hips and move into the Down-Face Dog.

6. Inhaling, come forward into the Up-Face Dog with your knees *off* the floor. Or, you can keep the knees on the floor, if that is easier for you.

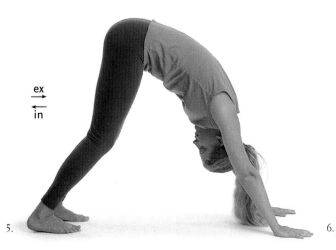

ex →
← in

in →
← ex

5.

6.

➤ *The Stick pose will build your strength in new areas. It does put pressure on your wrists, shoulders, and neck. If it gives you any discomfort or if you think it might, drop it from the sequence.*

➤ *If the Down-Face Dog is too difficult for you, substitute the forward bend part of the Cat stretch.*

➤ *You can combine the Standing Sequence (8.2) and this Kneeling Sequence without stopping the flow. Simply raise your arms in the standing position, bend forward placing your hands on the floor, and step back into the Down-Face Dog as you learned in 7.4. Then continue with the second sequence.*

3. Exhaling, bend forward moving your hips back and place your forearms on the floor.

4. Inhaling, move forward into the Cat arch, raising your head slightly.

in
→
←
ex

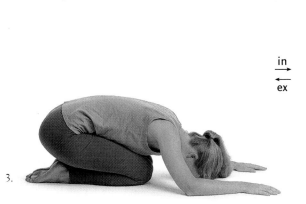

3.

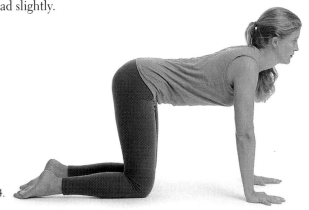

4.

---

7. Exhaling, lower down to the floor to the Stick variation, hands, chest, and forehead on the floor. You may want to relax the top of your feet to the floor in Up-Face Dog **(6)** and in the Stick **(7)**.

ex
→
←
in

7.

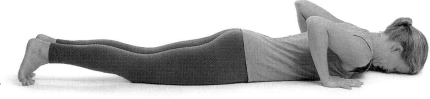

Now reverse the sequence.

6. Inhaling, go into the Up-Face Dog.

5. Exhaling, move back into the Down-Face Dog.

4. Inhaling, lower your knees and move into the Cat arch.

3. Exhaling, go back into the kneeling forward bend.

2. Inhaling, come up into the upright kneeling position with your arms overhead.

1. Exhaling, lower your arms.

• You can now begin the sequence again from here.

Repeat the sequence 1-4x.

8.4 UPWARD LEG AND ARMS STRETCH/BRIDGE COMBINATION

This final sequence includes a slightly new variation of the leg stretch and asks you to stay for two breaths in the Bridge pose.

1. Lie on your back with your knees toward your chest, hands comfortably over your knees.

2. Inhaling, stretch your legs up and bring your hands onto the floor behind you.

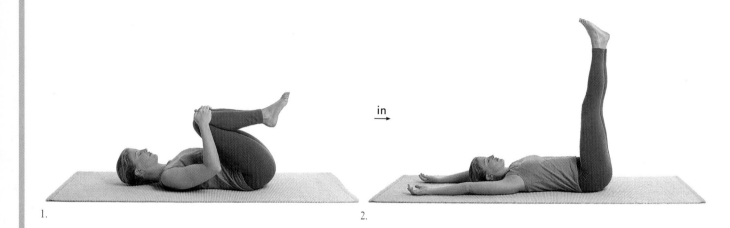

in →

1.

2.

5. Exhaling, bring both knees toward you.

6 & 7. Inhaling, place your feet flat on the floor, 6 to 18 inches apart, and go up into the Bridge arch.

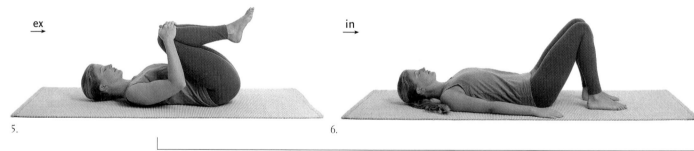

ex →

in →

5.

6.

Take one long inhalation as you move from the Knees to Chest pose to the Bridge arch **(5-7)**.

8 & 9. Exhaling, come down to the floor. After your hips touch the floor bring your knees to your chest.

Repeat the sequence 1-4x.

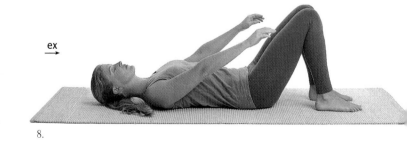

ex →

8.

Take one long exhalation as you move from the Bridge arch to the Knees to Chest pose **(7-9)**.

3. Exhaling, bend your right knee, and gently guide it toward you, right hand on your right knee, left hand on your right shin.

4. Inhaling, stretch your right leg up and bring your hands onto the floor behind you again.

• Repeat **(3)** and **(4)** with your other knee.

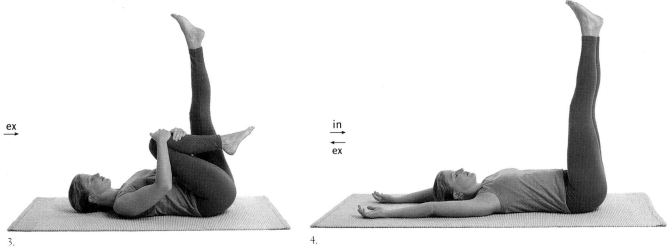

ex →

in →
← ex

3.

4.

Alternate legs.

7. Take two breaths as you stay in the arch.

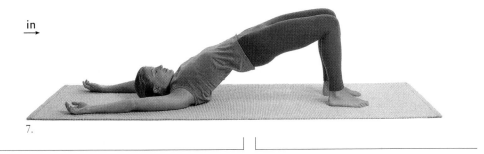

in →

7.

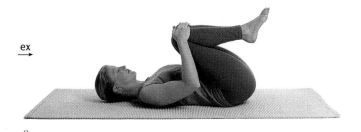

ex →

9.

You can practice all three sequences as one long sequence by making a smooth transition from the end of one sequence to the beginning of the next. In our classes, we often invent flowing vinyasas involving many variations–from standing to kneeling to sitting to lying down.

- Sit comfortably on a chair or pillow with your back straight, shoulders relaxed, and arms comfortably settled. Close your eyes.

- Take some easy breaths as you begin to turn your attention inward.

1. Now rest your hands lightly on your chest or abdomen. Take a few more breaths relaxing through your face and eyes.

2. When ready, place your hands on your knees, palms up.

1. Inhaling, raise your arms slowly and gently, bringing your hands to your heart or upper abdomen. Visualize bringing healing, caring energy inward. You may want to visualize bringing this energy to a certain area of your body. Stay for one or two easy breaths, taking your attention more and more deeply inward.

2. Exhaling, lower your head slightly as you slowly unfold your arms to bring your hands back to your knees with palms up. Release. Pause for several seconds, or take an easy breath, relaxing your face and eyes.

1. Inhaling, raise your head slightly and bring your hands to your chest or abdomen again.

- Continue the visualization pattern for 5 to 15 minutes.

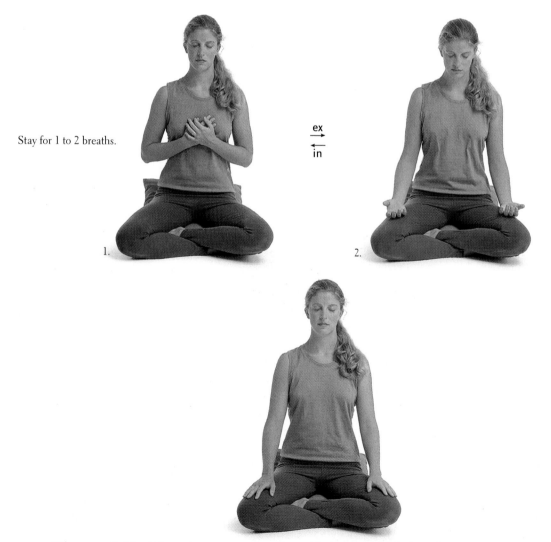

Stay for 1 to 2 breaths.

ex →
← in

1.

2.

When you finish, sit for as long as you like. Stay with the peaceful feeling from your visualization.

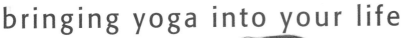

bringing yoga into your life

programs for every day

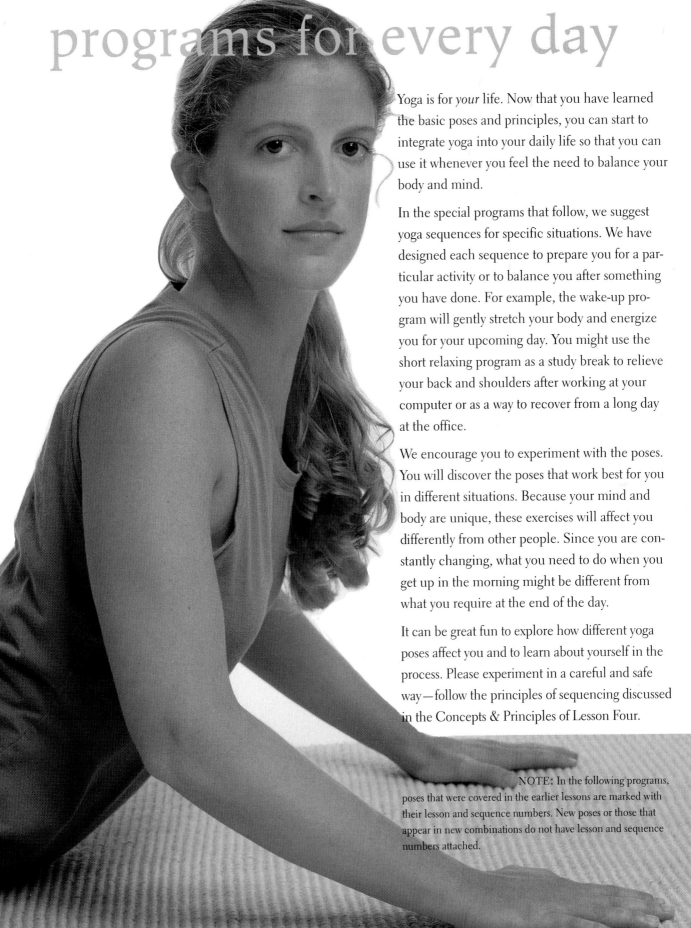

Yoga is for *your* life. Now that you have learned the basic poses and principles, you can start to integrate yoga into your daily life so that you can use it whenever you feel the need to balance your body and mind.

In the special programs that follow, we suggest yoga sequences for specific situations. We have designed each sequence to prepare you for a particular activity or to balance you after something you have done. For example, the wake-up program will gently stretch your body and energize you for your upcoming day. You might use the short relaxing program as a study break to relieve your back and shoulders after working at your computer or as a way to recover from a long day at the office.

We encourage you to experiment with the poses. You will discover the poses that work best for you in different situations. Because your mind and body are unique, these exercises will affect you differently from other people. Since you are constantly changing, what you need to do when you get up in the morning might be different from what you require at the end of the day.

It can be great fun to explore how different yoga poses affect you and to learn about yourself in the process. Please experiment in a careful and safe way—follow the principles of sequencing discussed in the Concepts & Principles of Lesson Four.

NOTE: In the following programs, poses that were covered in the earlier lessons are marked with their lesson and sequence numbers. New poses or those that appear in new combinations do not have lesson and sequence numbers attached.

yoga to wake up

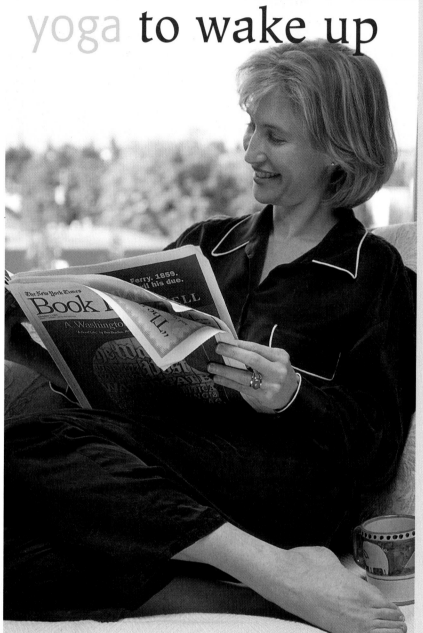

In the years after my two daughters Kate and Evelina were born, I, Margaret, would lie in bed not wanting to get up. The girls would be asleep, but I knew that they would soon be awake calling for my attention.

I needed to prepare for my day and gain energy slowly as a transition to being with them in a caring way. Yet it was hard for me to bring myself out of bed and practice yoga. Besides, if they heard me moving, they would be bound to wake up!

So, I would rearrange my covers, scoot down, and practice some "bed yoga." When I practiced this wake-up program it gave me the energy to practice a more vigorous program—if our daughters were *still* asleep—afterwards (which they usually were not). If they woke up, at the very least I would feel much better. Later in the day I would find time for a fuller program.

Now, years later, I admit I still do bed yoga at least one day a week! My program follows for you to use and adapt as you like.

1. Arm Raise with Leg Stretch

Lie comfortably in bed. Inhaling, raise your arms and slowly push your heels away from you, stretching your calf area. Exhaling, lower your arms and relax your feet and legs. You may like to bend one knee and place that foot flat on the bed. In this position, raise both arms and push out with the heel of your straight leg only.

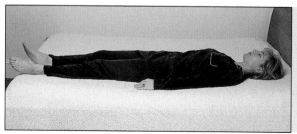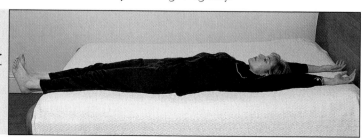

2. Upward Leg, Outward Arm Stretch (1.2)

Exhaling, bring your knee toward your chest. Inhaling, raise your leg and open your arms to the side.

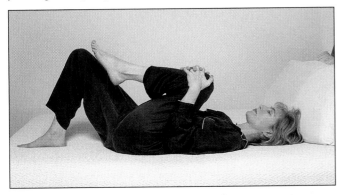

3. Bridge (1.3)

Inhaling, raise your hips and arms. Exhaling, lower them to the bed again. Of course this won't work on a waterbed!

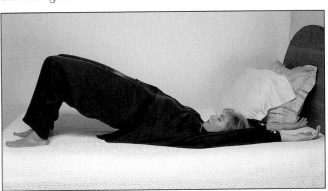

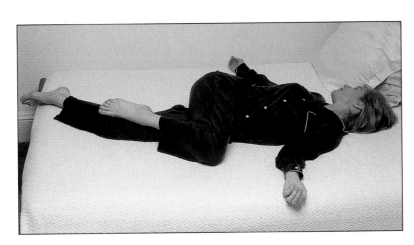

4. Lying Down Twist with One Knee Bent (3.9)

Exhaling, twist with one knee bent. Gently turn your head in the opposite direction. Inhaling, slowly bring your knee upright and turn your head back to center. Practice both sides equally.

5. Forward Bend, Side Stretch Sequence

Sit either cross-legged on the bed or sit on the side of the bed, with your feet well apart and flat on the floor.

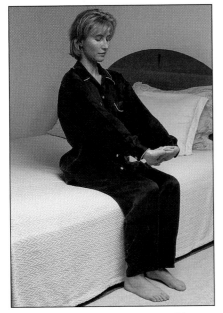

1. Interlace your fingers, palms out. If this is uncomfortable for you, keep your palms in.

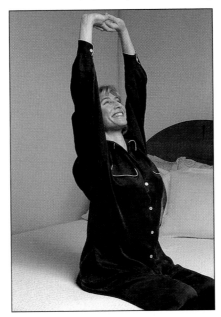

2. Inhaling, stretch your arms up overhead.

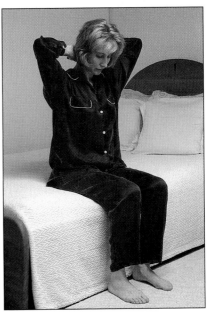

3. Exhaling, bend your arms bringing your interlaced fingers to or behind your head.

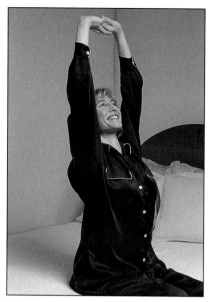

4. Inhaling, stretch up again.

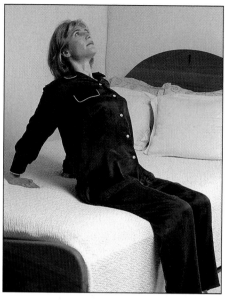

5. Exhaling, stretch your arms to the side and place your hands well apart behind you on the bed, palms down and fingers forward.

Inhaling, press your palms down gently as you open up through your chest. Keep your neck relaxed.

Exhale from your abdomen and keep your chest expanded.

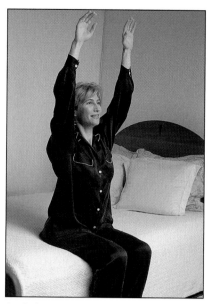

6. Inhaling, raise your arms.

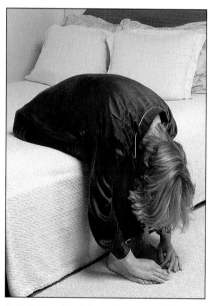

7. Exhaling, bend forward. Take one breath, arching as you inhale.

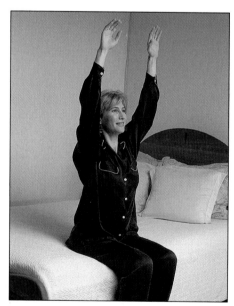

8. Inhaling, come up leading with easy arms and chest.

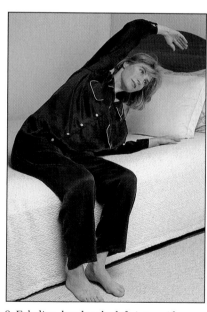

9. Exhaling, bend to the left, into a side stretch. Lean into your left forearm. Relax your head and right arm. Take one breath.

Inhaling, come up. Exhaling, stretch to the right. Take one breath.

➤ *You may also like to try doing this entire sequence with your eyes closed.*

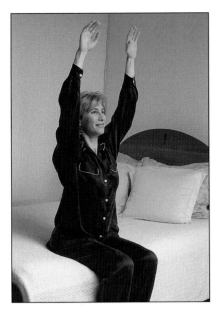

10. Inhaling, come up.

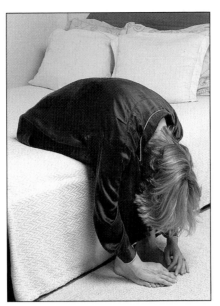

11. Exhaling, bend forward again. Take one or two breaths with or without arching as you inhale.

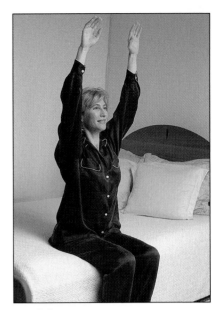

12. Inhaling, come up.

6. Seated Head Movements (3.11)

End your morning wake-up with gentle head movements. These will loosen any kinks in your neck from the night. Tip your chin up and down. Slowly turn your head to the left and right. Then move it back and forward again.

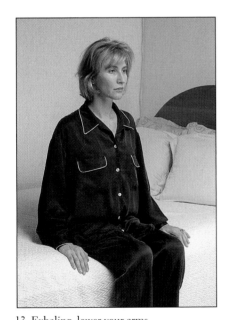

13. Exhaling, lower your arms.

Repeat the entire sequence or go on to Seated Head Movements.

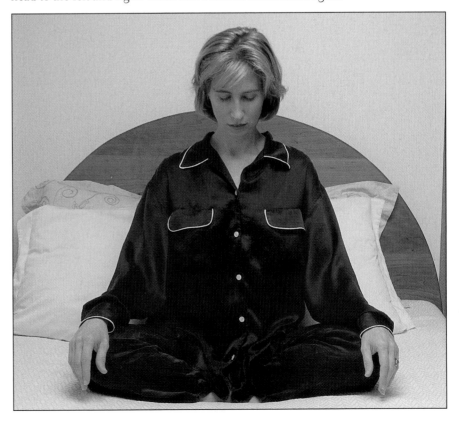

➤ *Remember to sit on a pillow or two to comfortably keep your knees lower than your hips.*

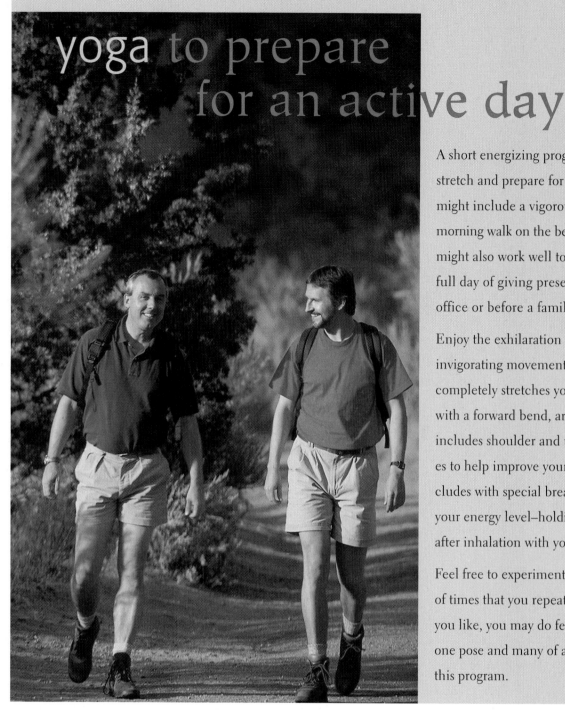

yoga to prepare for an active day

A short energizing program will help you stretch and prepare for an active day that might include a vigorous hike or a long morning walk on the beach. This program might also work well to vitalize you for a full day of giving presentations at the office or before a family reunion.

Enjoy the exhilaration of these simple, invigorating movements! This program completely stretches your legs and back with a forward bend, arch, and twist. It includes shoulder and upper back stretches to help improve your posture. It concludes with special breathing to increase your energy level–holding your breath after inhalation with your arms raised.

Feel free to experiment with the number of times that you repeat a given pose. If you like, you may do few repetitions of one pose and many of another pose in this program.

1. Standing Forward Bend (1.4 and 2.4) not pictured here.

Practice the Standing Forward Bend many times, keeping your arms well apart as you reach up. This will open up your chest. Take a breath or two in the bent-forward position, stretching your back. Inhaling, bend your knees more deeply and arch your back more. Exhaling, bend forward and straighten your legs somewhat to loosen your back and legs.

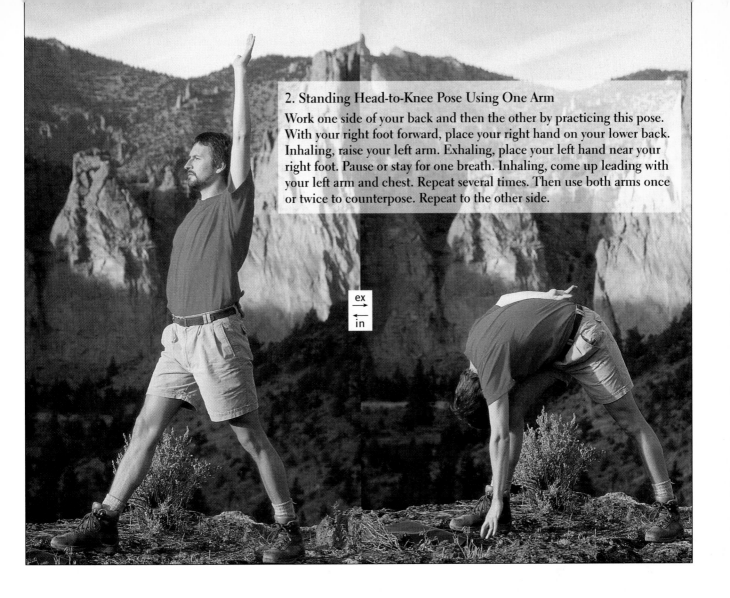

2. Standing Head-to-Knee Pose Using One Arm

Work one side of your back and then the other by practicing this pose. With your right foot forward, place your right hand on your lower back. Inhaling, raise your left arm. Exhaling, place your left hand near your right foot. Pause or stay for one breath. Inhaling, come up leading with your left arm and chest. Repeat several times. Then use both arms once or twice to counterpose. Repeat to the other side.

ex →
← in

3. Arm Stretch with Fingers Interlaced, and Standing Forward Bend Sweeping Your Arms

Repeat this standing stretch and energizing pattern several times.

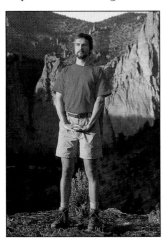

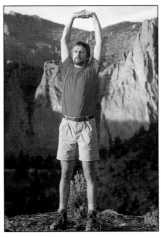

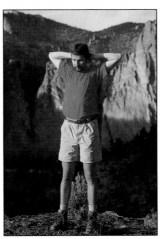

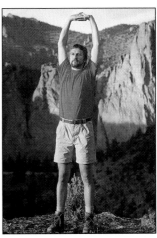

1. Stand with your fingers interlaced, palms out.

2. Inhaling, stretch your arms up overhead.

3. Exhaling, bend your arms, bringing your interlaced fingers to or behind your head.

4. Inhaling, stretch your arms up again, palms up.

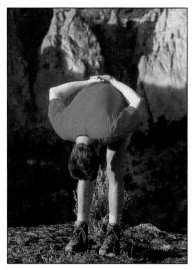

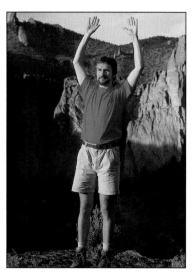

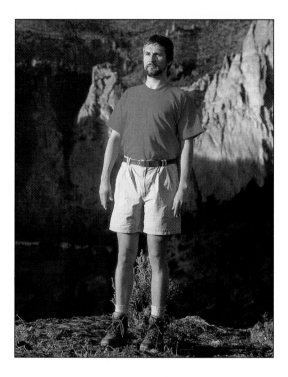

5. Exhaling, release your fingers, bend forward and sweep your arms to the side and onto your lower back. Pause or take a breath to stretch and release your back.

6. Inhaling, lower your hands toward the ground and come up leading with relaxed arms and chest.

7. Exhaling, lower your arms to the side.

4. Bridge, Guiding Knees Apart and Together

Lie on your back with your arms along your sides and feet well apart, flat on the ground. Place your knees together. Inhaling, raise your arms overhead and lift your hips, moving your knees well apart. Exhaling, guide your knees toward each other, staying up. Inhaling, part your knees again and raise your hips a little higher. Exhaling, lower down to the starting position, with knees together again.

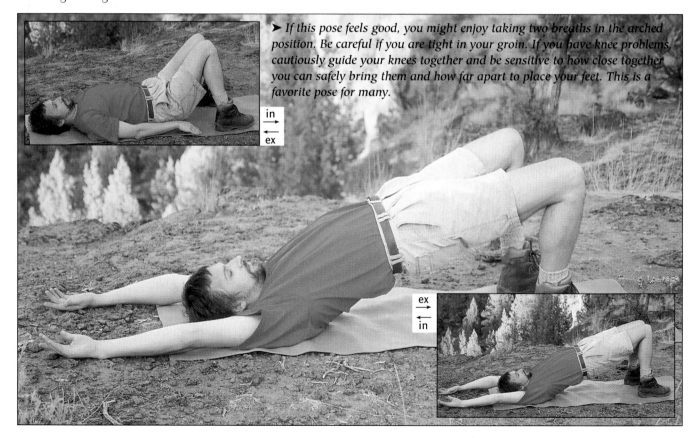

➤ *If this pose feels good, you might enjoy taking two breaths in the arched position. Be careful if you are tight in your groin. If you have knee problems, cautiously guide your knees together and be sensitive to how close together you can safely bring them and how far apart to place your feet. This is a favorite pose for many.*

in
←→
ex

ex
→
←
in

5. Lying Twist with One Knee Bent (3.9)

Now begin to cool down. Stretch out both sides of your back as you twist. Practice the twist several times on each side.

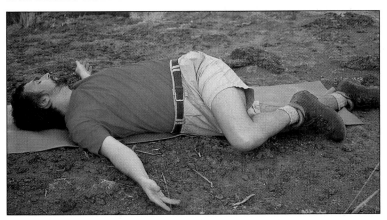

6. Upward Legs and Arm Stretch (2.9)

You will enjoy getting your legs up in the air after the standing poses. Practice a few repetitions of the Upward Legs and Arm Stretch. Notice if the previous poses have made you flexible enough to hold behind your knees and keep your legs up for 3-5 breaths. Exhaling, bend your knees slightly. Inhaling, straighten your knees. This variation wonderfully stretches tight and tired legs and back. In order to rejuvenate these areas, you might try this stretch again after your hike or a hectic day.

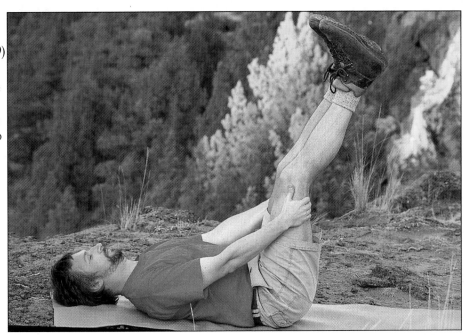

7. Arm Raise with Hold IN

Lie down and rest for several easy breaths. Then bring your arms alongside you, palms down. Inhaling, raise your arms overhead. Hold your breath for 2 seconds. Exhaling, lower your arms. With each arm raise, hold your breath for an additional second up to a maximum of six seconds. Continue for several more breaths, holding for the count that is most comfortable. Rest briefly and then sit up. Feel the energizing effects of holding IN.

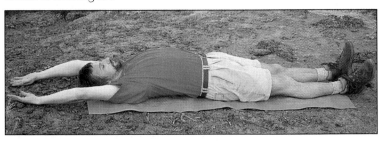

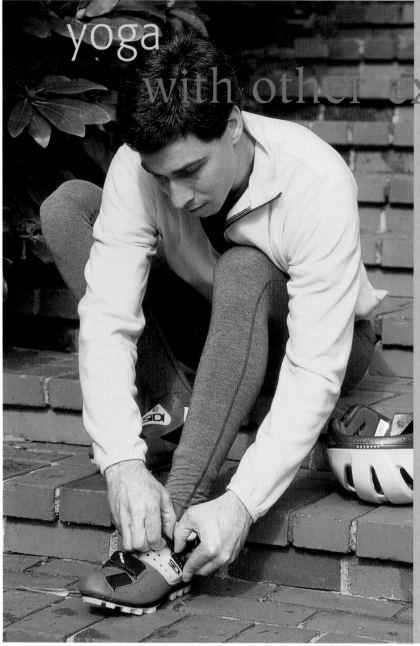

yoga
with other exercise

Running, cycling, softball, and swimming are a few of the many wonderful ways to get a cardiovascular workout. However, any exercise can strain or pull your muscles. Repeatedly practicing a given exercise will strengthen some muscles and neglect others.

You will be less likely to injure yourself, and you will perform better if you do yoga stretches before you exercise. Afterwards when your muscles have warmed up, yoga can keep them lengthened and relaxed and will gently realign your back and neck. Plus, yoga can help you be calm, alert, and focused—while you play and afterwards.

This program gives you a 7 minute warm-up before exercise and an 8 minute cool-down. When you practice this program, remember that over-stretching can contract the very muscles that you are trying to loosen. Stay relaxed and comfortable. Feel your slow, smooth breathing.

Enjoy your stretch!

before exercise—stretch and warm-up

1. Standing Forward Bend (1.4), (2.4)

First practice some simple forward bends dynamically to loosen up gently. Inhaling, bend forward. Then stay in the forward bend as you take a breath. Inhaling, bend your knees more deeply and arch your back. With each exhalation, straighten your legs more and feel the stretch. 4-6x.

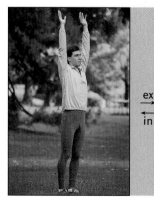
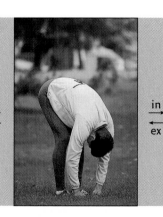
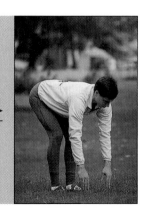

ex
in

in
ex

2. Standing Sequence (8.2)

Loosen up your back, hips, and legs with the standing dynamic sequence. (See Lesson 8 for the full sequence.) Work through the sequence continuously for 5 minutes. Stay and take a breath in the Forwards Bends, Twist, and Side Stretch if you like. This will increase your flexibility and warm all your major muscle groups before you work out.

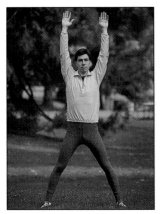

1. Inhaling, raise your arms.

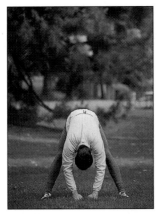

2. Exhaling, bend forward.

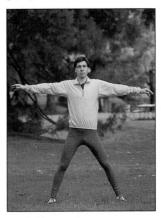

3. Inhaling, come up, raising your arms to your sides.

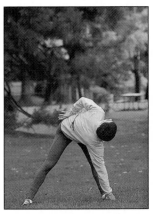

4. Exhaling, twist. Inhaling, come up. Exhaling, twist to the other side. Inhaling, come up.

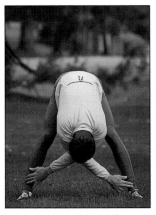

5. Exhaling, bend forward crossing your arms. Inhaling, come up.

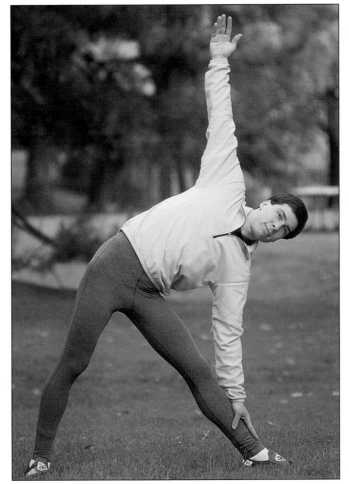

6. Exhaling, bend into the side stretch with your foot turned out. Inhaling, come up. Exhaling, bend to the other side. Inhaling, come up.

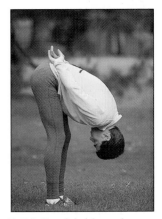

7. Exhaling, bend forward sweeping your hands onto your lower back.

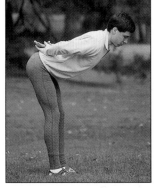

8. Inhaling, arch up part way. Exhaling, bend forward again. Inhaling, sweep your arms down and forward as you come up all the way.

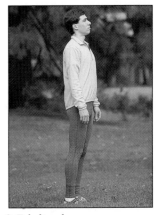

9. Exhaling, lower your arms.

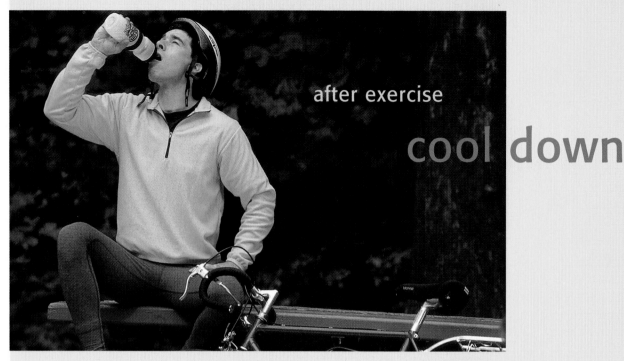

after exercise

cool down

After exercise, walk until your pulse comes down and you are breathing normally. Drink some water. While your muscles are still warm—at home, on soft level grass outside, or on a mat or carpet at the gym—cool down with this simple program.

1. Standing Forward Bend with Back Arching (1.4 and 2.4)—Using a Wall or Support

Stand with your back about 6 inches from a wall and your legs about shoulder width apart. Inhaling, raise your arms spreading them wide apart. Arch slightly. Tip your head slightly back, lightly touch the support with your fingertips, and open up through your chest and abdomen. Exhaling, bend forward and let your back stretch out. Take a breath in the forward position if you want. After several repetitions, try standing 8, then 10, or perhaps even 12 inches from the support, and repeat the pose. Arch and open up more. It feels great to open up gradually after vigorous exercise.

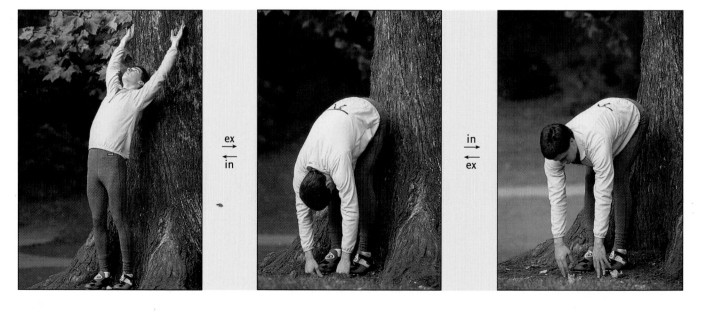

2. Upward Legs and Arms Stretch (2.9) Repeat 5-6x.

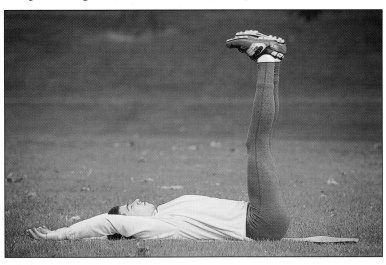

➤ *This cool-down program will take around 8 minutes. You will feel much better and your muscles will thank you.*

3. Bridge (1.3) Repeat 3-4 x.

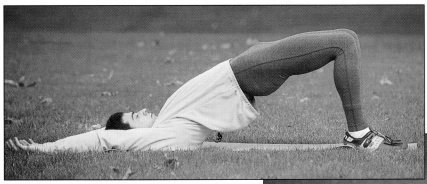

4. Lying Twist with One Knee Bent (3.9)
Repeat 3-4 x on each side.

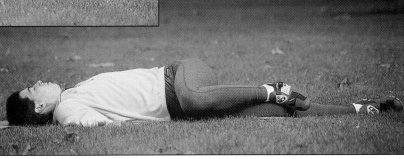

5. Knees to Chest Pose (1.5)
Finally, wind down by slowly bringing your knees into your chest as you exhale. Feel the stretch in your low back. Inhaling, guide your knees away from you with your hands and straighten your elbows. Repeat 4-5x with a slow relaxing breath pace.

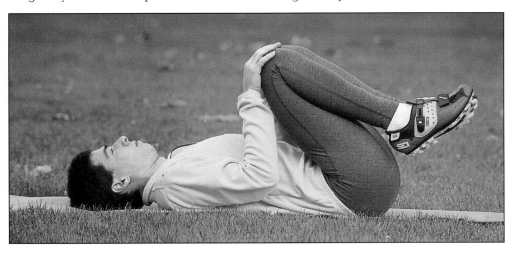

yoga

for a vigorous workout

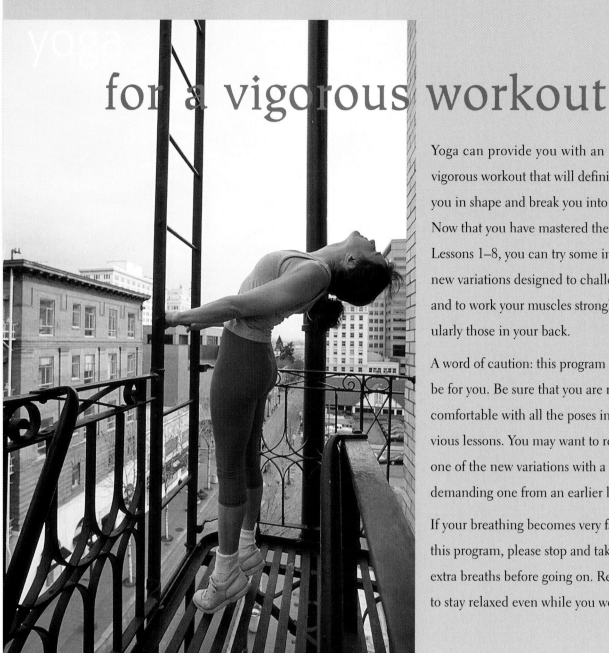

Yoga can provide you with an overall vigorous workout that will definitely keep you in shape and break you into a sweat. Now that you have mastered the poses in Lessons 1–8, you can try some interesting new variations designed to challenge you and to work your muscles strongly, particularly those in your back.

A word of caution: this program may not be for you. Be sure that you are really comfortable with all the poses in the previous lessons. You may want to replace one of the new variations with a less demanding one from an earlier lesson.

If your breathing becomes very fast during this program, please stop and take a few extra breaths before going on. Remember to stay relaxed even while you work hard.

1. Standing Forward Bend (1.4) and Standing Forward Bend with Leg Stretch (2.4)

Loosen up by doing the simple, dynamic forward bend. Then increase the work by holding for a breath in the forward bend and in the arch position. Repeat 6-8x.

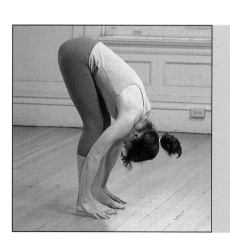

in
←
ex

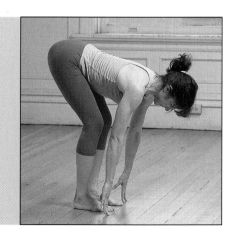

2. Triangle Twist to Side (3.3) and Triangle Twist to Center with Arm Movement

Practice the Triangle Twist to Side (3.3) to loosen up. Practice 2-3x each side.

Now practice the Triangle Twist to Center (4.4) adding some arm movement. From the twist position, inhale and sweep the hand on your hip down toward the floor and out in front of you. Arch and open through your chest and shoulders. Exhaling, twist more deeply, and sweep your arm to the side and back onto your hip. Inhaling, come up. Repeat 2-3x per side, alternating sides.

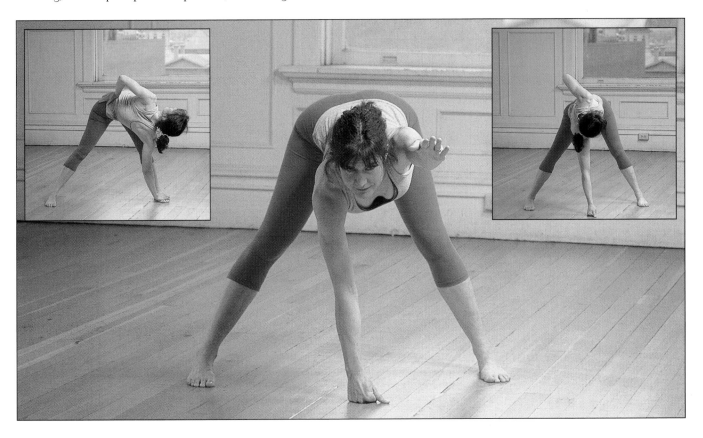

3. Standing Forward Bend Holding Dowel

Hold a standard-size dowel with your hands far apart. Keep your grip on the dowel light and relaxed. Practice the same forward bends you did in Step 1. Feel the added work holding the dowel. Make sure that you come up leading with your chest and the dowel. Keep your arms relaxed. Repeat 4-6x.

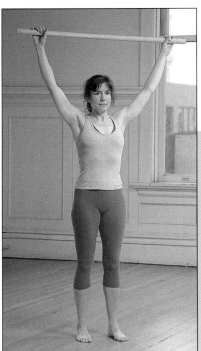

ex →
← in

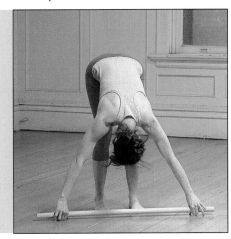

4. Standing Back Arch, Coming up Part-Way

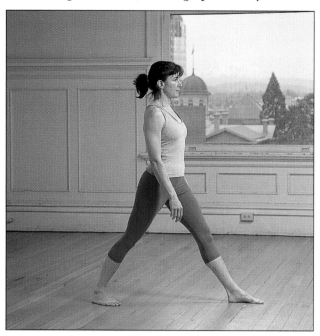

1. Stand with your left foot 2 to 3-1/2 feet forward. Turn your right foot out slightly.

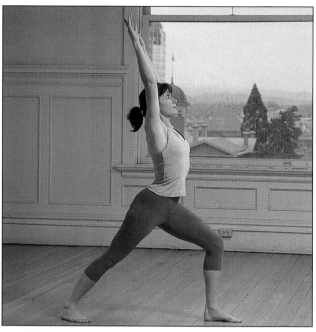

2. Inhaling, raise your arms from the front as you bend your front knee, and arch your back slightly.

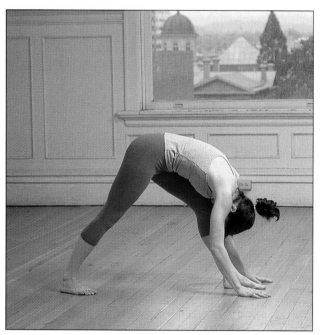

5. Exhaling, bend into the Head-to-Knee Pose, placing your hands on the floor to either side of your foot. Take an easy breath if you need to.

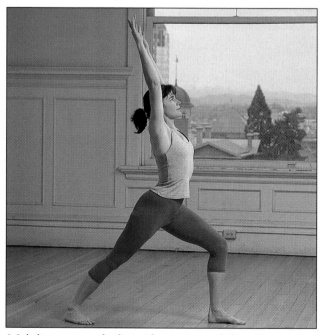

6. Inhaling, come up leading with your arms and chest. Keep your front knee bent and arch your back slightly. Exhaling, bend forward again and reverse the sequence. Continue this pattern until you want to come out completely.

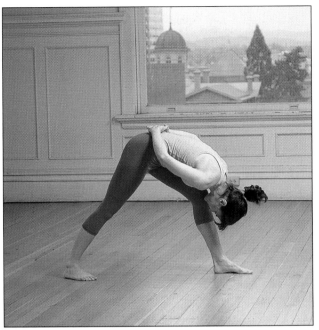

3. Exhaling, bend forward and lower your arms to the side, resting your hands on your lower back.

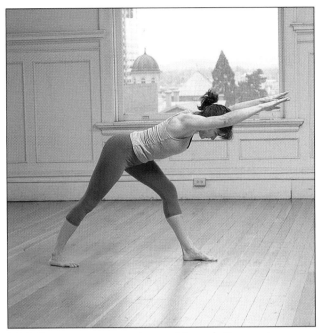

4. Inhaling, sweep your arms down and forward. Come part-way up, leading with your arms and chest.

To end the sequence:

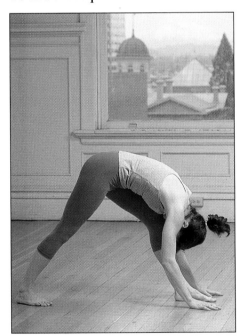

1. Simply exhale into the Head-to-Knee Pose.

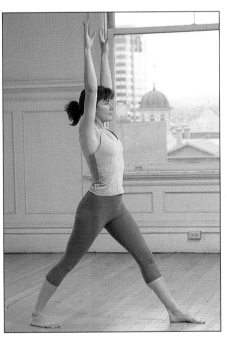

2. Inhaling, come up and straighten your leg.

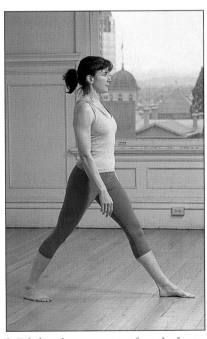

3. Exhaling, lower your arms from the front. Practice equally to each side.

Walk, sit, lie down, or go to the next pose.

5. Kneeling Forward Bend, Up-and-Down-Face-Dog/Strenuous Stick Sequence

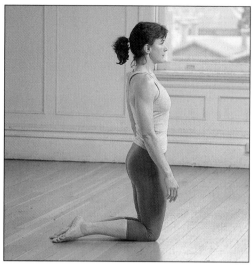

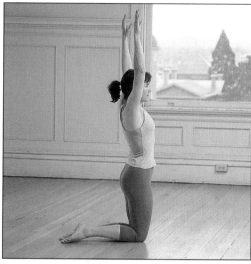

1. Kneel upright, with your knees slightly apart and your arms by your sides.

2. Inhaling, raise your arms from the front.

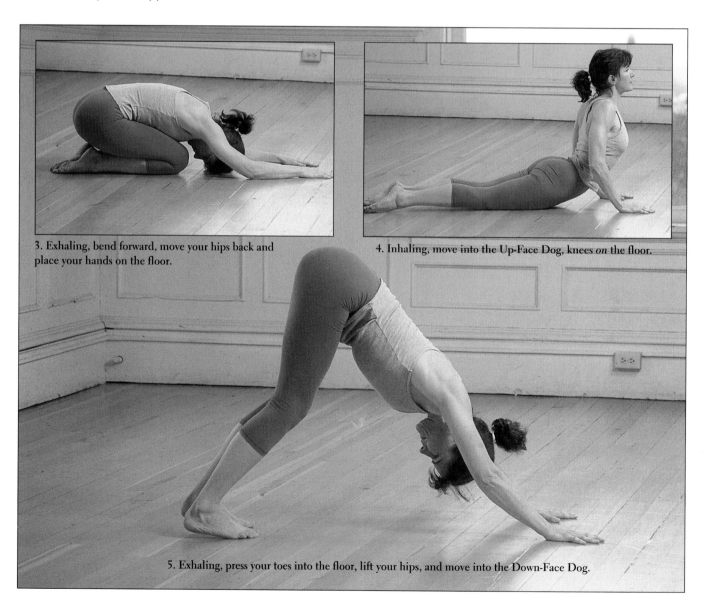

3. Exhaling, bend forward, move your hips back and place your hands on the floor.

4. Inhaling, move into the Up-Face Dog, knees *on* the floor.

5. Exhaling, press your toes into the floor, lift your hips, and move into the Down-Face Dog.

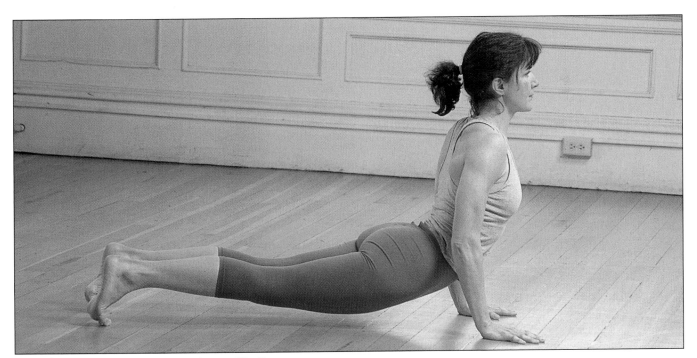

6. Inhaling, move into the Up-Face Dog, knees *off* the floor.

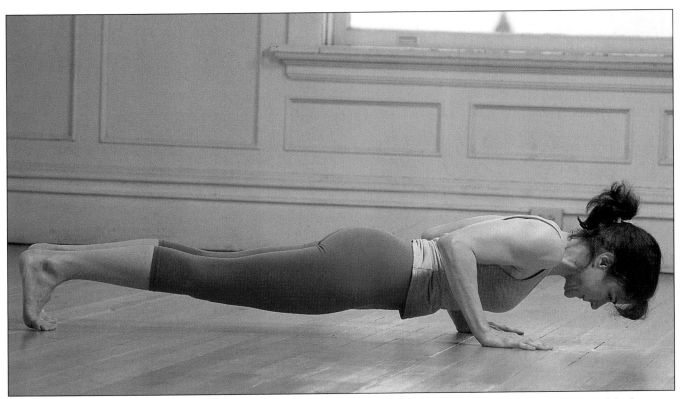

7. Exhaling, lower into a new Stick variation, bending your elbows back and bringing your abdomen, chest, and forehead in line just *off* the floor. Only your toes and hands are on the floor.

Now, reverse the sequence and go into the Up-Face Dog again with your knees *off* the floor. Continue to reverse the sequence until you come back to the initial kneeling position with your arms by your sides. Repeat the entire sequence (forward and reversed) 4-6x.

➤ *This is a challenging Stick variation. If you cannot keep your knees off the floor in the Stick and the Up-Face Dog, bring them onto the floor. If this is still too strenuous, use the Stick variation from the 8.3 sequence, dropping your hips, chest, and forehead to the floor.*

6. Upward Legs and Arms Stretch (5.2)

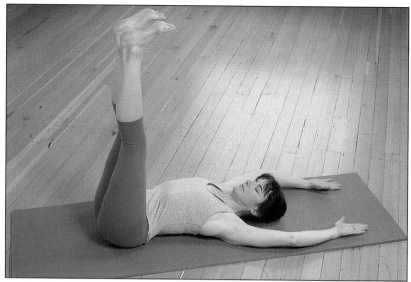

Counter the hard work you just did by releasing your low back, shoulders, and wrists in this pose. Work gently and slowly. Practice 5-6x.

7. Cobra/Locust with Arm and Leg Movements (7.10)

Now work hard again in this strong, back-strengthening pose. First practice the Cobra. Then move on to Locust raising your opposite arm and leg. Practice equally on each side. Finally, practice the Locust raising both your arms and legs. Practice each variation 3-4x. To make the poses yet more vigorous, stay up in the arch for a breath or two.

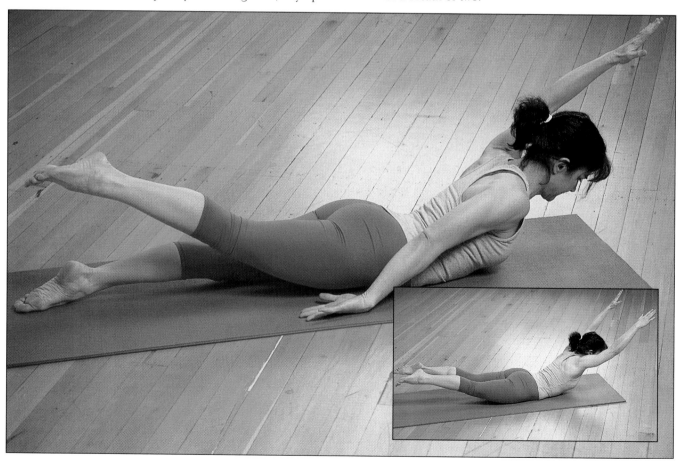

8. Knees to Chest (1.5) Repeat 3-4x.

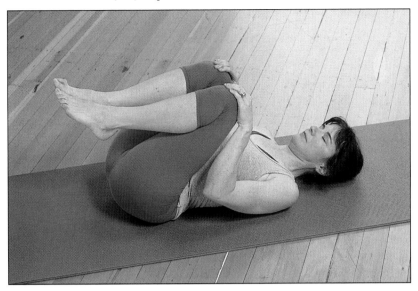

9. Seated Forward Bend

1. Sit on the floor with your legs in front of you, feet 8 to 16 inches apart and your back straight.

2. Inhaling, raise your arms from the front.

3. Exhaling, bend forward, arms relaxed. Take one breath.

2. Inhaling, come up, leading with your arms and chest.

Repeat 2-3x. Then try staying for 2-3 breaths, relaxing and stretching your legs and back as you release forward (3).

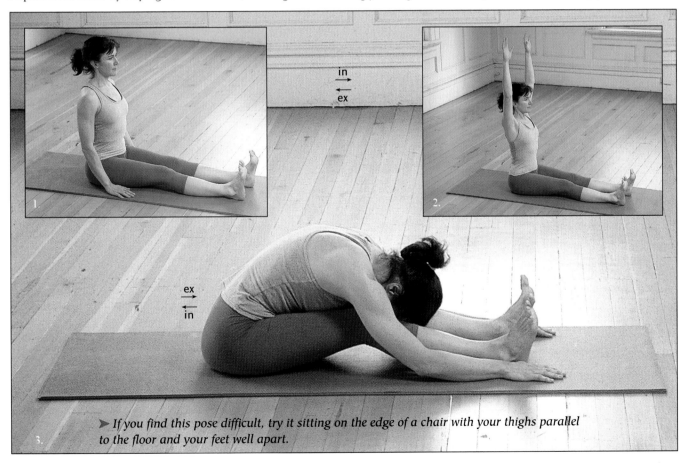

> *If you find this pose difficult, try it sitting on the edge of a chair with your thighs parallel to the floor and your feet well apart.*

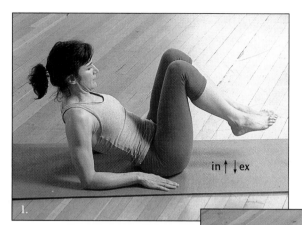

10a. One-Legged Boat

1. Sit with your elbows on the floor, palms down, knees bent. Place your heels several inches off the floor, feet together.

2. Inhaling, straighten your legs.

3. Exhaling, bring your right knee toward you.

2. Inhaling, straighten your right leg again.

3. Exhaling, bring your left knee toward you.

2. Inhaling, straighten your left leg again.

Continue with this pattern several more times with each leg.

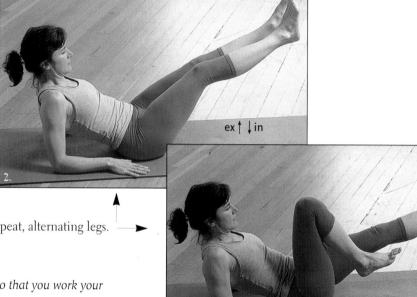

10b. Repeat with both legs. →

10b. Two-Legged Boat

1. Sit as in 10a.

2. Inhaling, straighten both legs.

1. Exhaling, bring both knees toward you.

10a. Repeat, alternating legs. →

➤ *Experiment to find the right angle so that you work your abdominals and thighs without straining your neck or back.*

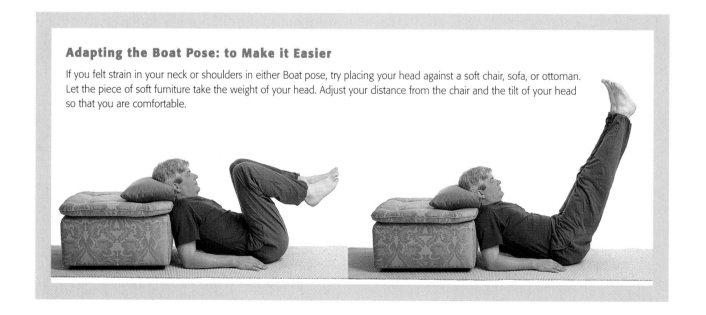

Adapting the Boat Pose: to Make it Easier

If you felt strain in your neck or shoulders in either Boat pose, try placing your head against a soft chair, sofa, or ottoman. Let the piece of soft furniture take the weight of your head. Adjust your distance from the chair and the tilt of your head so that you are comfortable.

Adapting the Boat Pose: to Make it More Challenging

If you want an additional challenge, try this Boat variation. Sit with all four limbs off the floor, balancing. Inhaling, raise both arms and legs. Exhaling, bring your right knee toward your chest. Alternate legs.

ex →

← in

11. Bridge, Arms Beside You

After contracting your abdominals and thighs in the Boat pose, you will find it a pleasure to stretch those areas in the Bridge pose. Inhaling, raise your hips. Keep your arms by your sides. For the first repetition, pause at the end of your inhalation. Then exhale and come down. The next time, stay in the arch for one breath.

Then stay for two breaths and then for three breaths. While staying, breathe deeply and smoothly, opening across your chest and keeping your arms and shoulders relaxed.

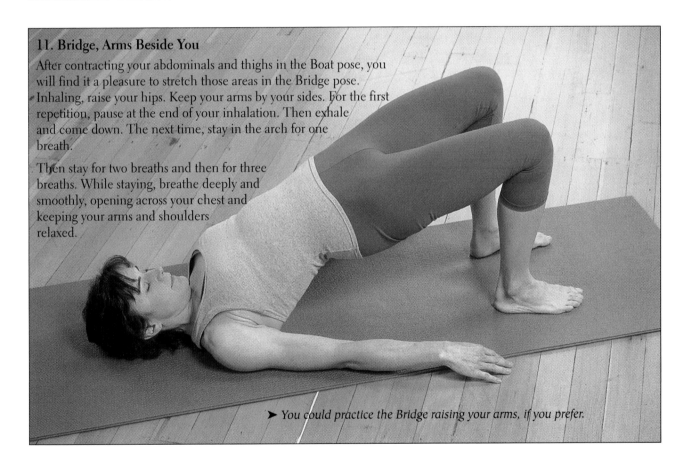

➤ *You could practice the Bridge raising your arms, if you prefer.*

12. Lying Eye and Face Relaxer (2.11)

Now relax for 10 to 20 breaths. Make your exhalation a few seconds longer than your inhalation. Think of softening in your face and eyes each time you exhale. Let your body release to the floor, and just feel the rhythm of your breath.

Then release control of your breath and breathe at a natural rate. Rest for two minutes, or as long as you like.

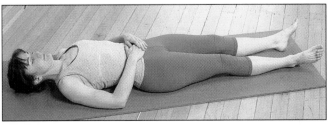

yoga
for a short relaxation

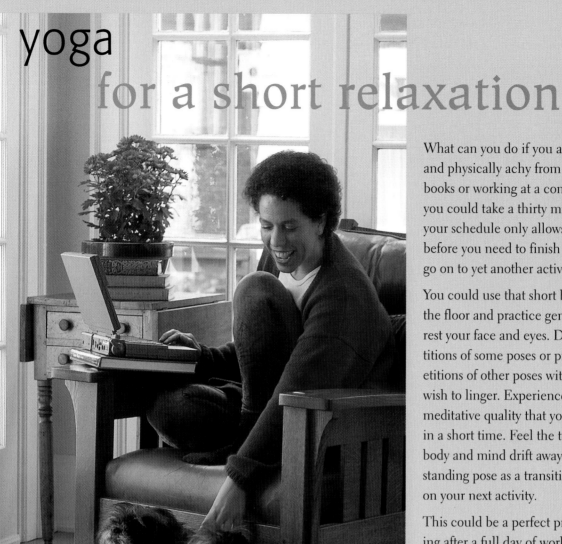

What can you do if you are mentally tired and physically achy from sitting over textbooks or working at a computer? You wish you could take a thirty minute nap, but your schedule only allows for a short break before you need to finish your project or go on to yet another activity.

You could use that short break to lie on the floor and practice gentle poses that rest your face and eyes. Do just a few repetitions of some poses or practice many repetitions of other poses with which you wish to linger. Experience the focused meditative quality that yoga can give you in a short time. Feel the tensions in your body and mind drift away. Then do a standing pose as a transition to focusing on your next activity.

This could be a perfect program for relaxing after a full day of work. Or you could use it on a Saturday at 4 pm after you have had a full week and a busy day. Stop. Acknowledge your fatigue and restore yourself with easy restful poses.

1. Arm Raise With Head Movement

Lie comfortably on the floor. Inhaling, raise both arms. Pause. Exhaling, lower your arms, turning your head gently to the left. Pause. Inhaling, raise your arms, turning your head to face the ceiling. Exhaling, lower your arms, turning your head gently to the right. Relax through your face and eyes. Continue this pattern, alternating sides.

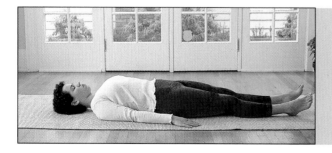

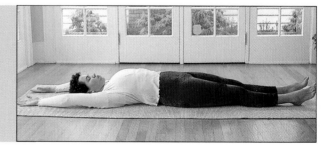

in
←
ex

2. Combination Leg Lift and Leg Stretch

Lie with your left foot flat on the floor, your right leg extended straight, and your arms at your sides with palms down. Inhaling, raise your arms to the floor over your head. Exhaling, lower your arms as you raise your right leg slowly to a 90 degree angle to the floor. Continue your exhalation as you bend your right knee and bring it comfortably toward you, placing your left hand on your right knee and your right hand on your shin. Inhaling, raise your arms to the floor over your head and slowly straighten your right leg to a 90 degree angle. Continuing the same inhalation, bring your leg back to the floor again. Repeat this pattern several times—open with each inhalation, close with each exhalation. Then change legs. Rest briefly.

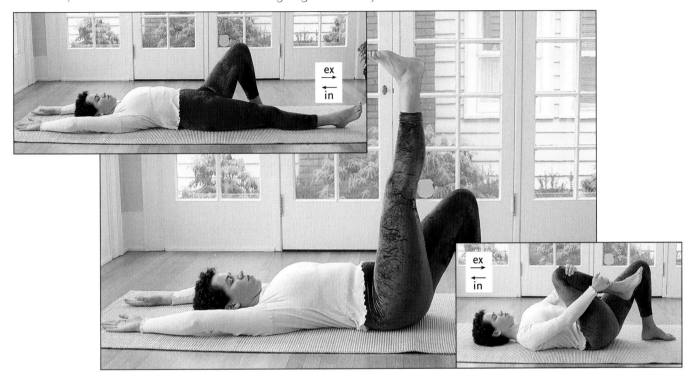

3. Bridge, Arms Beside You

Keep your arms comfortably settled beside you, palms down. Inhaling, feel your chest expand as you lift your hips. Exhaling, feel your abdominals gently contract as you slowly come down. You may want to take a breath in the arched position.

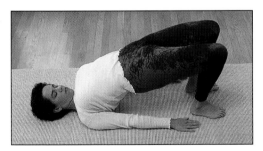

4. Lying Twist with Both Knees Bent (1.6)

Exhale slowly into the twist. After your exhalation stay there, holding your breath out for 2-5 seconds. Relax into the twist. Then, inhaling, bring your knees back to the upright position. Continue, alternating sides.

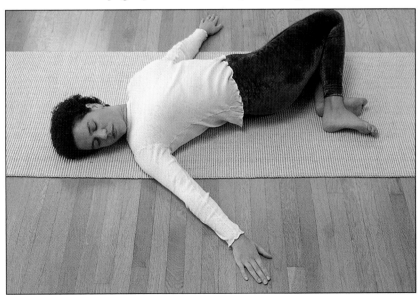

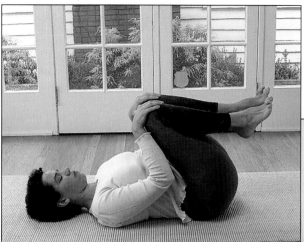

5. Upward Legs and Arms Stretch (2.9)

You might enjoy getting your legs up in the air once more after hours of sitting. Practice several repetitions. If you are flexible you can stretch more by pushing your heels way from you slightly at the end of your inhalation. For even more stretch, you might like to try bringing your legs 1, 2, or 3 feet apart.

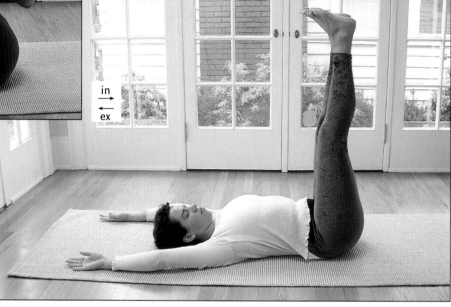

in →

ex →

6. Seated Head Movements (3.11)

This pose should release neck strain from driving in heavy traffic or from working at your desk all day. Exhaling, lower your head. Relax into the stretch, letting go through your neck, face, and eyes. Inhaling, raise your head slowly, stretching in the front of your throat. Repeat 2-3x. Then turn your head from side to side 2-3x. End the sequence by lowering and raising your head again, to realign your neck 2-3x. Then sit quietly and enjoy the relaxed feeling within you.

You may want to end here or finish with the next standing pose sequence.

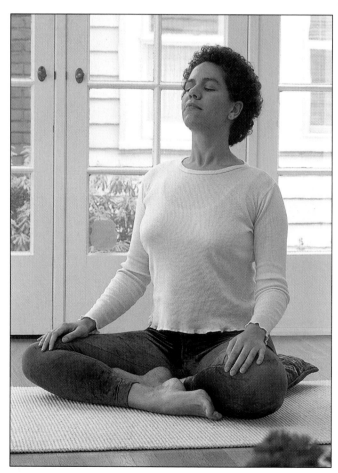

7. Standing Forward Bend, Opening Arms Out to the Side

Now that you have gained some relaxed energy, you may want to use a standing pose as a transition to your next activity. This will refresh, stretch, and energize you before you go back to study, make dinner, or go out for the evening.

Stand and place your hands between your lower abdomen and chest. Inhaling, bring your arms out to the side, expanding your chest. Exhaling, bend forward and hold your toes, ankles, or calves. Inhaling, bend your knees more and arch your back. Lift your head slightly. Exhaling, bend down. Inhaling, come up with your arms out from your shoulders and open up through your chest. Exhaling, place your hands on your front and stay briefly. Is one repetition enough, or would you like to do another, or perhaps many more?

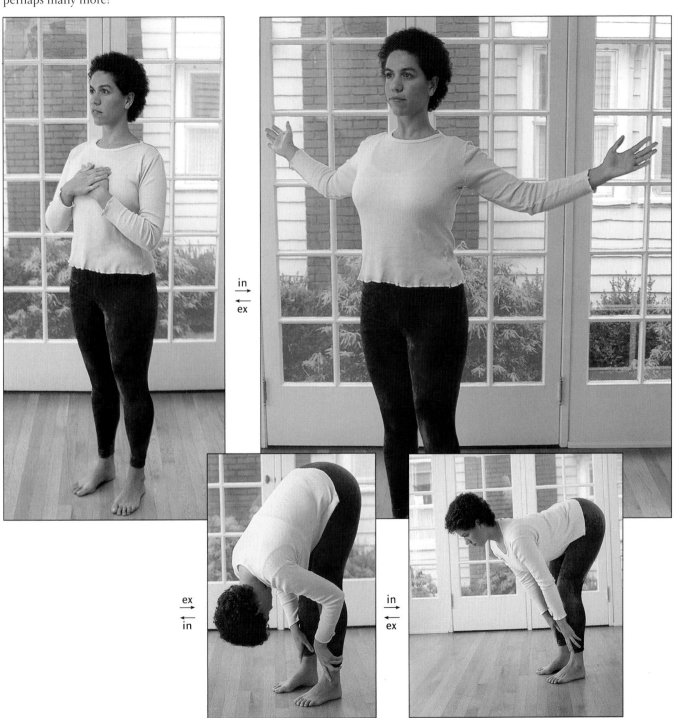

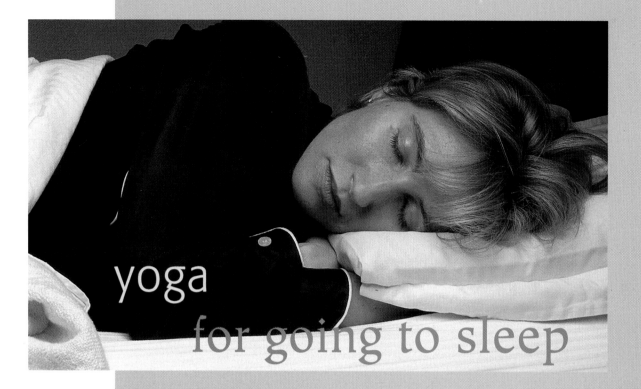

yoga
for going to sleep

Both of us teach until late at night. Often one of us starts teaching around 4:30 pm and ends at 10:30 pm. We come home, have a light bite to eat, and talk together about the day. It is often difficult to wind down and get to sleep before midnight.

If I, Martin, have difficulty getting to sleep, I do many slow repetitions of the Standing Forward Bend—down and up, down and up. I use an easy inhalation and focus on a longer exhalation. However, what works for me does not always work for Margaret.

I, Margaret, use the same easy inhalation and long exhalation as Martin, but I bend forward to the bed. With my hands on the bed, I take one, two, or three breaths. I bend my knees and arch as I inhale, and I straighten my legs a bit and stretch down as I exhale. I finish by lying down on my back, hands on my abdomen, to do some breathing—drawing my attention more and more inward. After a while I roll over onto my side and place a pillow under my head and perhaps another between my knees. I continue slow easy abdominal breathing, relaxing my forehead, facial muscles, and eyes. I draw my attention even more deeply inward by visualizing a deep, rich, velvety-purple color. Before long I am inhaling about 3 seconds and exhaling about 3 seconds, deeply relaxed, falling fast asleep.

These practices and poses work for us. They may work for you, or you may need something different. Some people might need to work off some restless, tense fatigue by starting with a Dynamic Standing Sequence (8.2). Many of our students say that they sit in bed and use the Caring Breath (5.12), relaxing through their face and eyes, until they lie down to sleep. Experiment freely. The effects of breath and movement are different for everyone. What works for you?

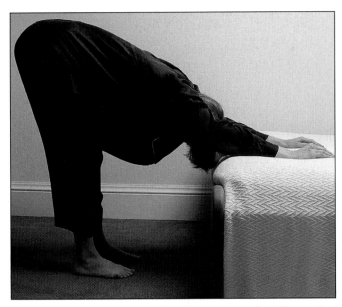

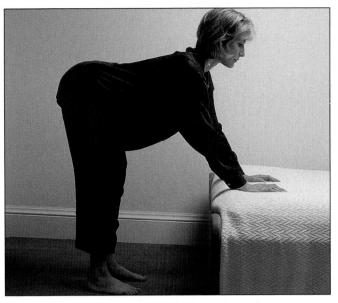

Exhaling, relax your back with a few easy Standing Forward Bends to the bed.

Inhaling, arch gently with your hands on the bed.

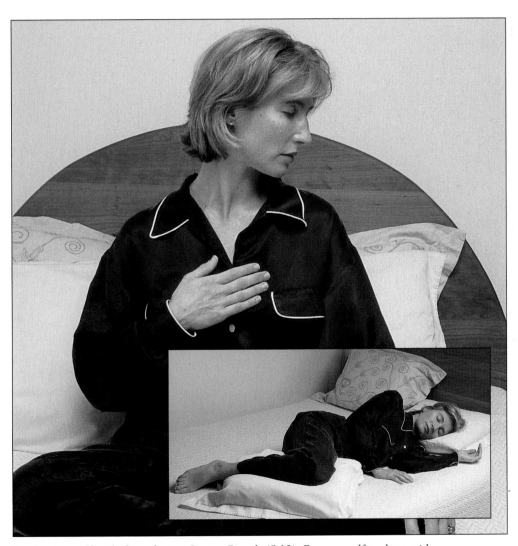

Soothe yourself with the calming Caring Breath (5.12). Put yourself to sleep with visualization and slow breathing.

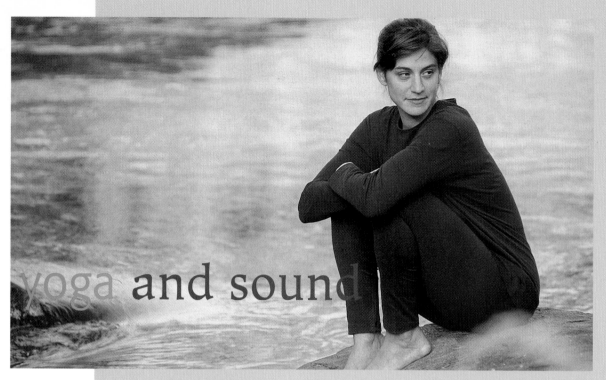

yoga **and** sound

Like the soothing sound of waves breaking on a beach or water rippling in a stream, our breath continuously sings in us. Soothing vibrations—sounds—can help us to release our tensions.

Adding simple sounds to some poses can multiply the benefits of your yoga practice. Sound can help you increase your inner focus and awareness. It can help you feel more in harmony with yourself and the world around you. It can give you a deep sense of quiet. Sound can still your mind.

Combining sound with yoga poses particularly helps people with breathing problems and speech difficulties. Not only does the force of sound naturally regulate and lengthen your breath, it also breaks up muscle tension in your face, mouth, jaw, and rib cage. Carol Fulwiler Jones, 42, is a psychotherapist in private practice. She tells us: "I had a Temporal Mandibular Joint (TMJ) problem for many years. That is the joint where your jaw is attached to your skull. I had to wear a device in my mouth at night to keep from grinding my teeth down. Then I learned to do some yoga poses using sound. Within a week my jaw relaxed to the point that I didn't have to wear the device at night. Now when I use sound with my yoga practice and make a conscious effort to relax my jaw muscles, the tension is completely relieved."

About eighty percent of the women in our pregnancy classes consciously use sound at some point during labor. Some use the sound as a "controlled expression of pain." Women like to make the sounds "ah", "ma", and "o" during painful contractions. Others students use sound with painful kidney stones, intense menstrual cramps, gas pains, or even in an ambulance coping with a painful hip fracture.

You can work with sound to examine your breath and your mental and physical state. Are you able to maintain the same pitch and volume throughout a movement? Is the sound steady or does it waiver or pulsate? Can you keep it from dying down at the end of a movement? If the answer is "no" to any of these questions, you could benefit by working on your breath. Practicing yoga with sound is one way to do that.

The following lesson is an introduction to yoga and sound. If you enjoy it, you might ask a teacher to introduce you to the many other ways of using sound—loud, soft, 'silent', multiple sounds, and visualization with sound. It is a fascinating exploration.

In this program, you will make a simple, drawn out, "AH" ,"O", or "OM" sound while exhaling. Most people are comfortable with the "AH"and "O" sounds. They bring your attention downward and inward. For some people, the "OM" sound is useful. They think of it as an affirmation of their true self, the source of energy and mental clarity within.

Let the sound come out freely from the very bottom of your abdomen. Don't be shy. You may want to try really singing out or try softening the sound. What's the difference? One way may be more appropriate than the other depending on your mood, the movement, and where you are practicing. Just relax and let the sound flow.

a practice with sound

In each of the following poses, practice 2-3x *without* sound and then 3-4x with a long, steady "AH", "O", or "OM" sound. You can experiment with the volume of the sound, making it loud, medium, or soft.

1. Tree (4.1)

Relax and get in touch with your breathing by doing simple arm movements. Exhaling, let your arms float downward with the sound. Use the full length of your exhalation to complete the movement and sound. Remember to relax your elbows and shoulders.

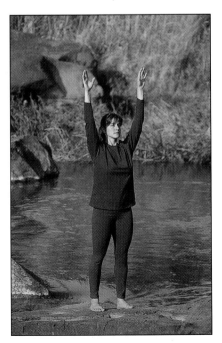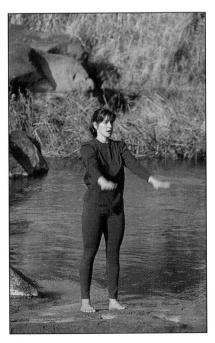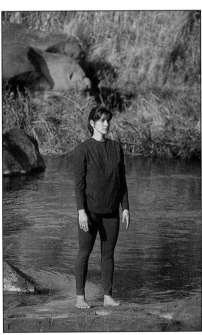

AHHHH....as you Exhale.

2. Standing Forward Bend (1.4)

Use sound as you exhale and bend forward. Pause and feel a quiet space at the end of your exhalation.
As you lower your arms after each repetition, bring the sound inward by silently thinking it.

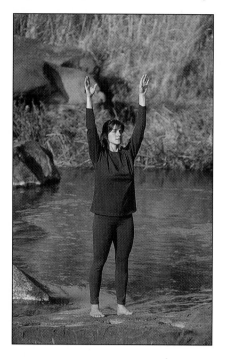 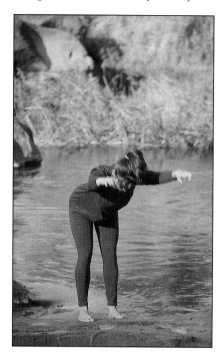 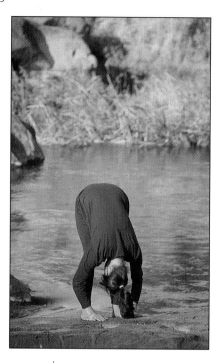

AHHHH....as you Exhale.

3. Triangle (2.3)

Listen to the "AH" resonate as you turn first to one side and then to the other. Do you notice a difference in your breath and the sound between the two sides? Can you steadily maintain the volume of the sound to the end of this movement? If one side of your body is tighter than the other, you will notice that your sound will differ going to the left compared to the right.

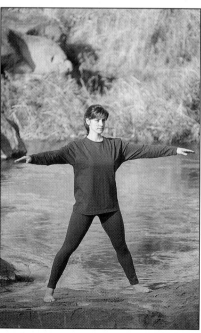 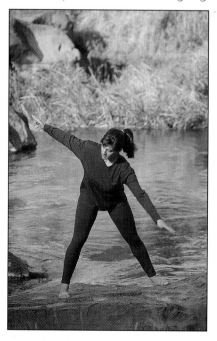 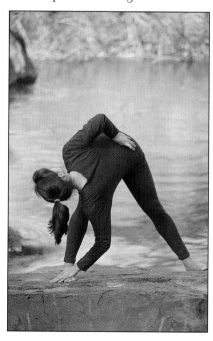

AHHHH....as you Exhale.

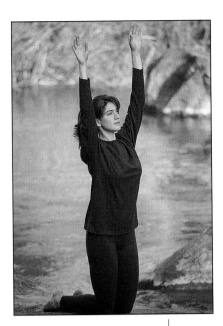

4. Kneeling Forward Bend/Cat (3.8)

Exhaling in the Forward Bend and in the Cat, make a sound of your choosing. You can try making an internal silent sound or a vocal sound as you lower your arms.

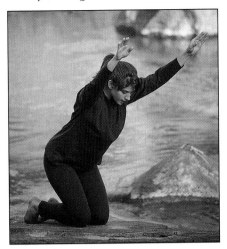
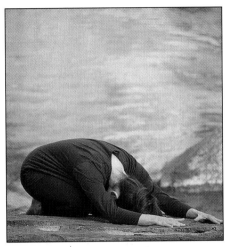

Oooo....as you Exhale.

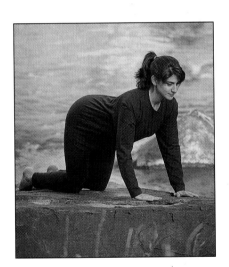
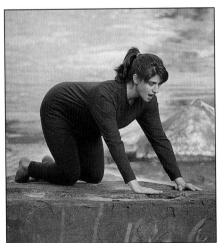
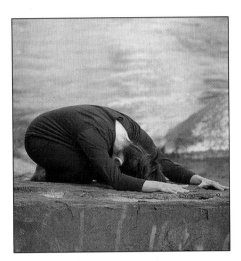

Oooo....as you Exhale.

5. Upward Legs and Arms Stretch (2.9)

Finally move *without* sound. Rest your voice and enjoy the stillness.

Note: Sound does not work well when you are lying on your back or are upside down.

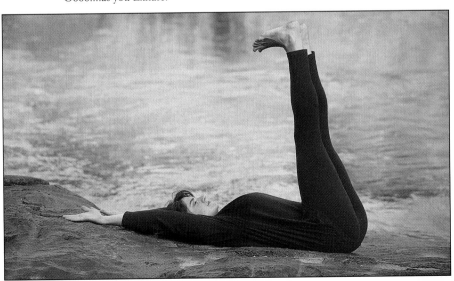

6. Seated Sounding

Sit on a pillow or a chair with your eyes closed. Take a few easy breaths. Feel the peaceful rhythm of your breathing. Then place your hands on your abdomen or chest. Keep your arms and shoulders relaxed.

Choose the sound "AH", "O", or "OM". Inhaling, move your arms comfortably out to the side. Exhaling, use the sound as you bring your hands slowly back to your front. Stay for an easy breath just thinking the sound as you exhale. Continue this pattern of arm movement and sound for some time.

Sing out! Experiment with drawing out the sound. The more uninhibited you can be about singing out, the more relaxing, centering, and energizing the sound will be. Fill your mind and your body with sound.

When you finish, place your hands on your chest, abdomen, or knees. Sit for a few minutes. Stay with the feeling of the sound.

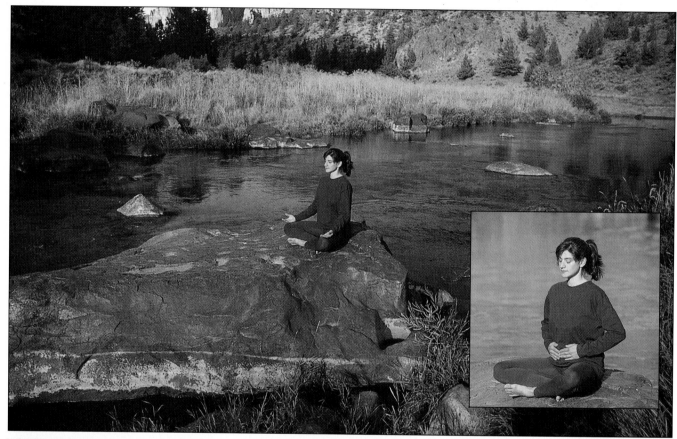

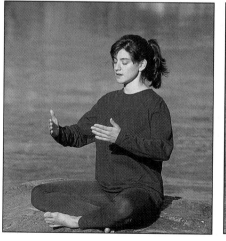

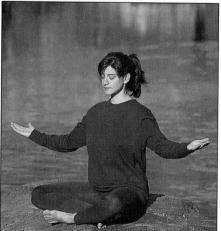

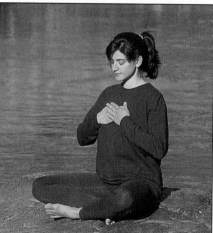

Oooo....as you Exhale.

yoga
as a deeper meditation

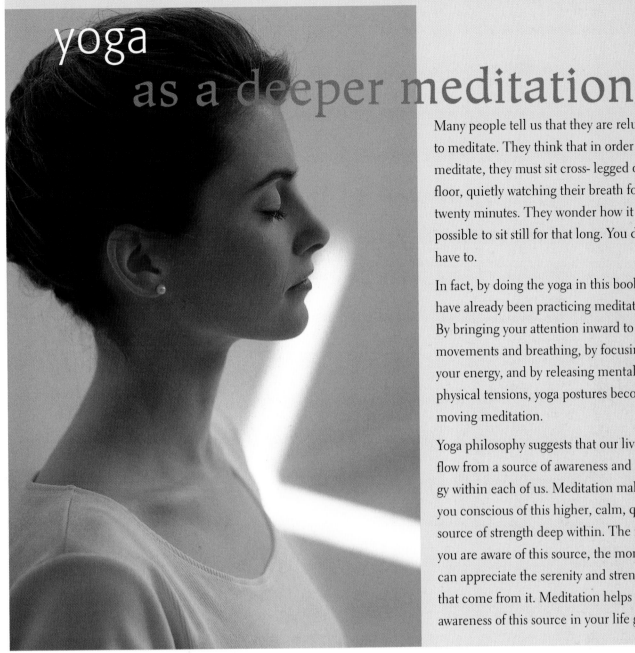

Many people tell us that they are reluctant to meditate. They think that in order to meditate, they must sit cross-legged on the floor, quietly watching their breath for twenty minutes. They wonder how it is possible to sit still for that long. You don't have to.

In fact, by doing the yoga in this book, you have already been practicing meditation. By bringing your attention inward to your movements and breathing, by focusing your energy, and by releasing mental and physical tensions, yoga postures become a moving meditation.

Yoga philosophy suggests that our lives flow from a source of awareness and energy within each of us. Meditation makes you conscious of this higher, calm, quiet source of strength deep within. The more you are aware of this source, the more you can appreciate the serenity and strength that come from it. Meditation helps your awareness of this source in your life grow.

The process of yoga meditation begins when you decide to take a break from your daily activities and turn your attention inward. In the process, you will look at your true nature. You may ask: "Who am I? What am I doing? Why am I doing it?"

Ideally, everybody should receive an individualized meditation from a competent teacher. To be most effective, meditation simply cannot be generic. Choosing a meditation is an art. It must suit your background, temperament, interests, and ability to focus. Since we know that it is not possible for everyone to have a teacher, in this lesson we suggest a simple practice along with ideas to help you develop your own meditation.

To do yoga meditation, you need to focus on some object that helps you go inside yourself. The object can be something in nature such as a leaf or flower, a tree, rushing water, the sound of a bird, or the sun. It can be a person who embodies the spiritual qualities that you would like to attain, such as Christ, the Buddha, or a great teacher. It could even be a vision of yourself free of problems or free of the characteristics that interfere with your relations with others.

The object of your meditation can be a picture or a color. You might use a *mantra* or a vocal or silent sound, such as "Om" or "Amen." Or you might focus on the feeling associated with a word like compassion, trust, strength, or truth. Try repeating a phrase or prayer. Before your practice, you might enjoy reading a meaningful passage from a book and then meditate on that.

Freely experiment to see what is most useful. What feels right for your meditation may well up from somewhere deep within you. What intuitively feels best?

You might begin by meditating for just a few minutes. Or perhaps you will be comfortable sitting for fifteen minutes right away. The length of time is less important than the quality. People often ask when they should practice. Morning is usually best, but the main thing is to meditate when you don't have to look at the clock for half an hour.

Never force yourself to meditate. It is a waste of time and is not productive. Some days you might set out to do a half hour meditation and find that instead you need thirty minutes of strong yoga poses or twenty minutes of easy poses and ten minutes of lying down restful breathing. You can even do your meditation after a long *asana* practice.

Where you meditate is also important. Ideally you will have already found a quiet, clean, and comfortable place where you regularly practice yoga. Going to that spot should quiet your mind. After you have established a yoga habit, that spot will evoke a feeling of serenity.

Ideally, you plan your meditation first, as you would a Shoulderstand program. You prepare for the Shoulderstand, practice it, and do the counterpose. Then you come out in a slow transition that allows you to move on to what you need to do next in your day. The same is true for a meditation practice.

To begin, warm up with simple yoga poses to make your body comfortable, begin to regulate your breathing, and quiet your mind. When you have gained a feeling of relaxed energy, you are ready to sit in meditation.

Next, sit comfortably erect and focus on your breathing to steady your mind.

Then, think about what kind of object might help you move toward a deeper awareness. Go more deeply inward, breathing slowly and focusing on your chosen object. Feel or experience the object in whatever way you can. Then let go of thinking about it. Allow it to fill your mind until you become mentally almost one with it. This is the heart of meditation, the part that will bring you closer to your deepest self.

Finally, gradually make a transition to the next activity of your day. Sit quietly or do a simple yoga pose. Going from your meditation room to the kitchen, office, car, or child should not be a jolting experience.

Meditation does not always happen easily. You will be distracted at times. Our minds, like the wind, are hard to control. Sometimes we think about everything but what we are trying to focus on. When this happens, simply notice the distraction, accept it, and gently bring your attention back inward.

The following is an example of a meditation for you to try. It will give you an idea of how to create a meditation practice of your own. Experiment. It takes a long time, as well as lots of reflection and practice to find a useful, highly personal meditation. A teacher who knows you can be a great help. Your practice will change as you grow and change through your meditation. Enjoy the lifetime journey.

preparing your body for meditation

First, practice a few yoga poses. They will stretch and relax your muscles so that you can sit more comfortably in meditation, without being distracted by your body.

1. Standing Forward Bend, Hands on Front Sequence

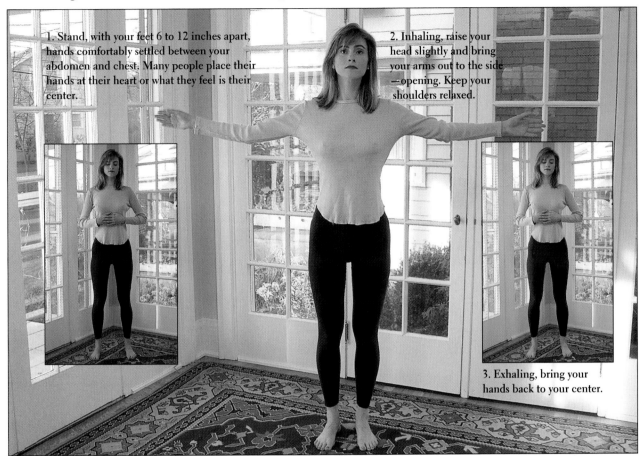

1. Stand, with your feet 6 to 12 inches apart, hands comfortably settled between your abdomen and chest. Many people place their hands at their heart or what they feel is their center.

2. Inhaling, raise your head slightly and bring your arms out to the side —opening. Keep your shoulders relaxed.

3. Exhaling, bring your hands back to your center.

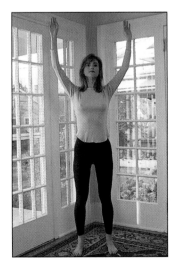

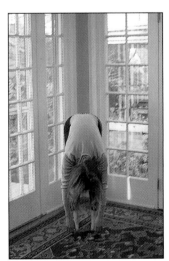

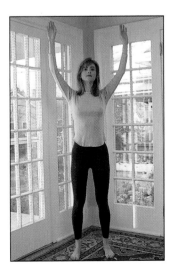

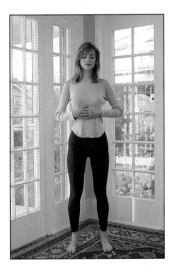

4. Inhaling, reach up with your arms well apart. Arch slightly.

5. Exhaling, bend forward. Pause at the end of your exhalation or stay and take one breath.

6. Inhaling, come back up into a slight standing arch.

7. Exhaling, lower your chin and place your hands over your center. Stay briefly. Repeat 3-4x.

2. Kneeling Forward Bend/Cat (3.8) or Up-Face Dog (4.6) Sequence

Practice 2-3x gently.

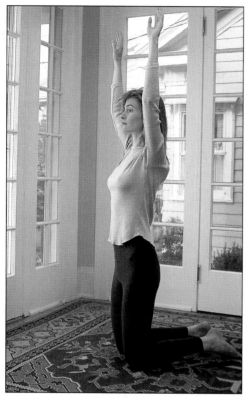

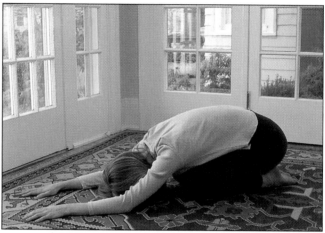

2. Exhaling, bring your hips back towards your feet, placing your hands on the floor.

1. Inhaling, raise your arms.

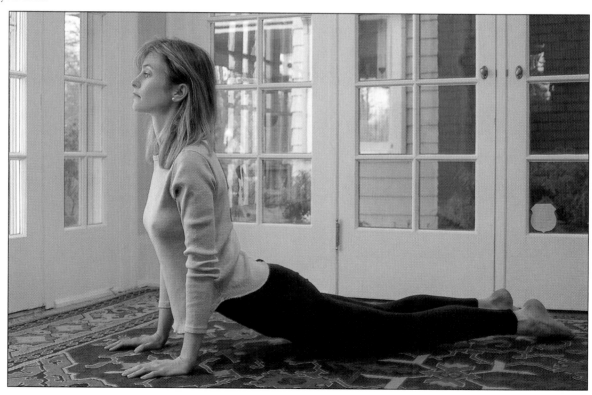

3. Inhaling, move forward into Up-Face Dog. Or, if you like, you can move forward into Cat. From Up-Face Dog or Cat reverse the sequence.

3. Upward Legs and Arms Stretch (2.9)

Stretch your legs before sitting for meditation. Exhaling, guide your knees toward you. Inhaling, stretch your legs up and bring your arms to the floor behind you. Repeat 2-3x.

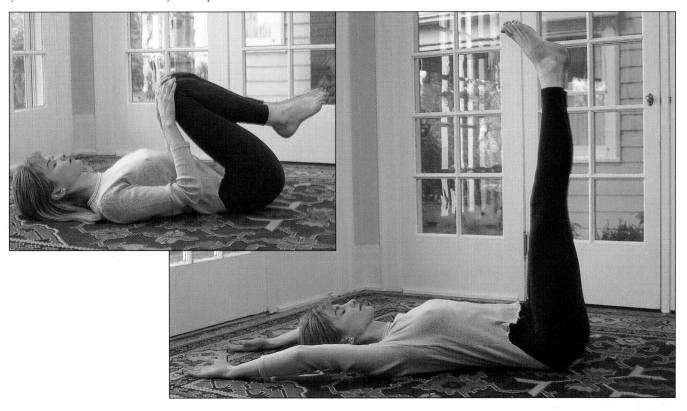

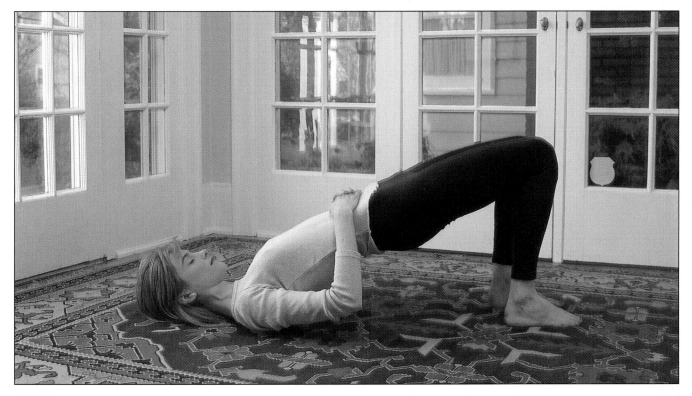

4. Bridge

Place your hands comfortably on your abdomen, arms and shoulders relaxed. Inhaling, raise your hips into the Bridge pose. Stay for one breath. Exhale down. Stay for one breath. Continue 4-5x. Rest briefly.

a meditation practice

Sit comfortably on a chair or pillow. Focus on your breath. Breathe easily and naturally. Gently keep your attention on your breath to quiet your mind and thoughts.

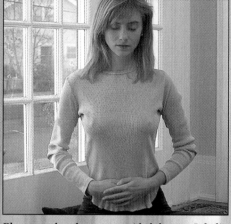

Place your hands on your mid-abdomen. Inhaling, visualize vital healing energy coming into you. Take 6-8 breaths. Allow that energy to expand throughout your body.

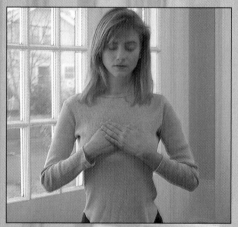

Place your hands over your heart. Begin to visualize trust, trust in yourself, and perhaps trust in a source deep within you. Stay with this feeling of trust for 6 to 8 breaths. Feel a contact with something strong and quiet within.

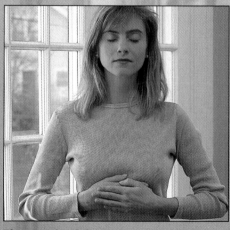

Place your hands between your navel and your heart. Breathe comfortably. Simply feel the flow of your breath. Feel your breath merging into a still presence.

transition back to your day

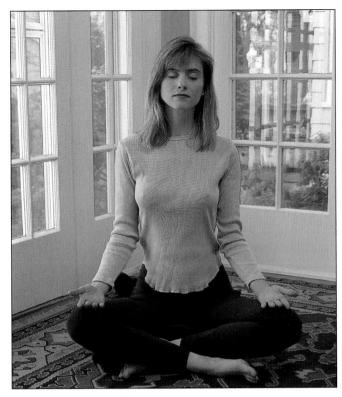

When you are ready to come out of meditation, briefly place your hands on your knees, palms up. Continue to feel the effects of your meditation.

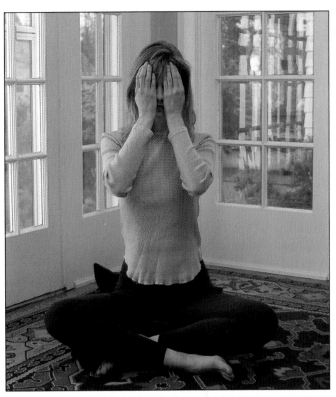

Some people like to palm their eyes for a few breaths. Keep your elbows, hands, and head comfortably relaxed.

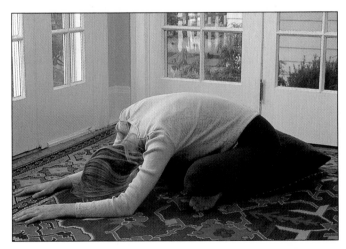

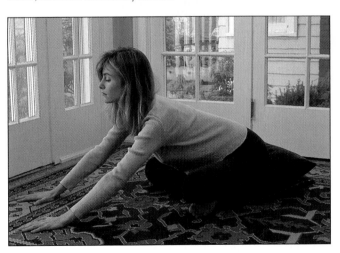

Exhaling, bend forward. You can try keeping your legs crossed or extend them as you bend over. If you have been sitting in a chair, simply bend forward, relaxing toward your knees and letting your arms come down toward the floor. Take a few breaths. As you inhale, straighten your arms. Exhaling, bend down again.

When you are ready, open your eyes.

Finally, walk quietly around your room for a minute or so. Try to take the feeling of yoga with you into your life.

acknowledgments

We would like to thank the many people who have advised and encouraged us to write this book. First and foremost we are grateful to our teacher Sri T.K.V. Desikachar for his insight, his enormous breadth of knowledge, his sensitive creativity, and his 'heart-to-heart' teaching in the tradition of his father, T. Krishnamacharya.

We are grateful to our students, who helped us to understand which yoga teachings work and how to best explain them.

Many friends have read parts or all of this book, giving us valuable suggestions. Among them: Sonia Nelson, Sherry Baker, Mary Lou Skelton, Dorothy Conlon, Albert Franklin, Larry Payne, Diane Thomas, Dolphi Wertenbaker, and Jane Young.

It has been a great pleasure working with everyone at Rudra Press. We are grateful to Monica O'Neal, who had the imagination to make this book far more useful than we had conceived, and who has skillfully and unstintingly refined and shaped it; Bill Stanton, who directed the art, did the design and layout, and made this a visually beautiful book; Lubosh Cech, who worked diligently at the lesson compositions; Ellen Hynson, who did the seamless fine tuning of the text, and to Karen Kreiger, who helped in so many ways.

We thank Barry Kaplan (together with his assistant Kenneth Ross) for his wonderfully sensitive, clear photography and for his patience in working with us. Thank you to Judy Kuniansky, photographer and friend, who took most of the black and white photographs.

We also would like to thank the many people who consented to be interviewed for this book: Pam Durban, Art Harris, Carol Fulwiler Jones, Richard Keenlyside, Ellen Mickiewicz, Rachel Newberry, Kim Papastavridis, Bobbi Patterson, Don Payne, Katie Teel, Miles Wilson, and several others whom we did not have space to quote.

We thank all of those who gave generously of their time to model for this book: Jennifer Albert, Lubosh Cech, Sasha Goldstein, Karen Kreiger, Akana Ma, Robin Mesch, Gary Peurasaari, Steve Reznick, Deborah Thrall, Laura Washington, and especially Shannon Brake and Edie Heintz, who flew to Portland for the photography sesssions.

We would like to thank Pat Marcus, Charlene Ball, and Lisa Hinely for their help in typing.

Martin would like to thank Bruce Pemberton, Louis McCleod, Joseph Reid, and Perry Treadwell for their patient support. Margaret thanks Ginny Green who helped more than she will ever know.

We want to express our gratitude to Martin's father, William Curtis Pierce, who made it possible for us to write this book.

Finally, we thank our daughters, Kate and Evelina, for their patience with us as we devoted many hours to writing.

The authors and the publishing team give their gratitude to Swami Chetanananda and the Nityananda Institute for their very generous help and support, which made the production of this book possible.

the authors

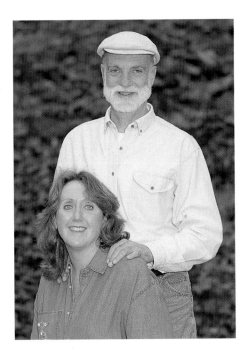

Margaret and Martin Pierce direct the Pierce Program in Atlanta, Georgia. Martin began practicing yoga in 1968 while teaching political science at New York University. In 1972, he met T.K.V. Desikachar and studied with him for a year before returning to the U.S. where he began teaching yoga in Atlanta, Georgia.

Margaret Pierce first practiced yoga in 1971. In 1974, she and Martin traveled to India to study with Desikachar. When they returned to Atlanta, they established the Pierce Program. Since then, they have studied with Desikachar almost annually in India, Europe, or the United States. Since 1983, Martin has taught yoga in Emory University's Health and Physical Education Department.

Martin graduated from Yale University, has an M.A. from the University of Wisconsin, and has done graduate work in political science at the University of Minnesota. Margaret graduated from Marietta College and studied for two years at the Institute of European Studies in Vienna, Austria.

THE PIERCE PROGRAM

The Pierce Program offers classes in yoga exercise, breathing, meditation, and the philosophy and psychology of yoga. It also trains teachers in these areas.

Margaret Pierce founded and directs the Pierce Pregnancy Program. Its classes teach yoga-based exercises and breathing, inform students about the childbirth process, and function as support groups for women. Margaret teaches special workshops on childbirth and delivery to pregnant women and their partners.

For information on programs and classes, please contact:

The Pierce Program
1164 N. Highland Avenue, N.E.
Atlanta, Georgia 30306
(404) 875-7110

about Rudra Press

We hope that you enjoy Yoga for Your Life. *Rudra Press publishes books, audios, and videos on yoga, spirituality, meditation, health, and healing with sound and music. Our mission is to provide powerful and practical works that guide our customers to the discovery of harmony, inner balance, and well-being.*

For more information on Rudra Press's complete line of products or to request a free catalog, please call or fax toll-free

1-800-876-7798 or fax **1-800-394-6286**.

Rudra Press
P.O. Box 13390
Portland, OR 97213

products of related interest:

BOOKS

Yoga for Body, Breath and Mind A.G. Mohan

Stretch and Surrender:
A Guide to Yoga, Health, and Relaxation for People in Recovery
Annalisa Cunningham, M.A.

The Breath of God Swami Chetanananda

Will I Be the Hero of My Own Life? Swami Chetanananda

The Open Moment Swami Chetanananda

Healing Imagery & Music Carol Bush, L.C.S.W.

Secrets of Natural Healing with Food Nancy Appleton, Ph.D.

The Natural Healing Cookbook Bessie Jo Tillman, M.D.

The Simple Path to Health Kim Le, Ph.D.

AUDIOS

Hatha Yoga in Motion Nityananda Institute

Meditation: A Guided Practice for Every Day
Swami Chetanananda

VIDEOS

Lilias! Yoga for Better Health Lilias Folan

Lilias! Alive with Yoga: Beginner Lilias Folan

Lilias! Alive with Yoga: Intermediate Lilias Folan

Lilias! Energize with Yoga Lilias Folan

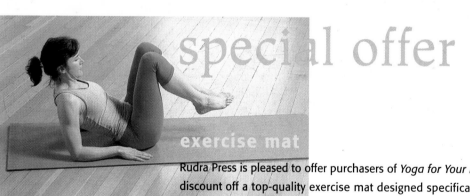

special offer

exercise mat

Rudra Press is pleased to offer purchasers of *Yoga for Your Life* a 20% discount off a top-quality exercise mat designed specifically for yoga practice by Hugger Mugger, a manufacturer of yoga products. The Tapas® Mat comes in purple, pearl grey, or lapis blue.

To order and receive your 20% discount, please call Hugger-Mugger at

1-800-473-4888.

Be sure to mention where and when you bought *Yoga for Your Life* in order to receive this special offer.